The Ultimate Dr. Sebi Cookbook

Alkaline Transition Made Easy with 1800+ Days of Healthy, Practical and Delicious Recipes. Master the Art of Alkaline Nutrition with Everyday Recipes for High Vitality

Angela Harper

Copyright

The contents of this book may not be reproduced, duplicated, or transmitted without the written permission of the author or publisher. Under no circumstances shall the publisher, or the author, be held liable or legally responsible for any damages, compensation, or monetary loss due to the information contained in this book. Either directly or indirectly.

Legal notice: This book is copyrighted. This book is for personal use only. You may not modify, distribute, sell, use, quote, or paraphrase any part or content of this book without the consent of the author or publisher.

Disclaimer: This book is intended for informational purposes only. The information in this book is not a substitute for the advice, diagnosis, or treatment of a medical professional. The theories and practices described are based on Dr. Sebi's teachings and the author's research. The author assumes no responsibility for any adverse effects or consequences resulting from the application of the information provided.

Index

The Ultimate Dr. Sebi Cookbook ... 1

Alkaline Transition Made Easy with 1800+ Days of Healthy, Practical and Delicious Recipes. Master the Art of Alkaline Nutrition with Everyday Recipes for High Vitality ... 1

PREFACE ... 7

Introduction to the alkaline diet ... 7

   Origins and Philosophy ... 7

   Core Principles of Alkaline Eating ... 8

   Common Misconceptions Clarified ... 10

CHAPTER 1: UNDERSTANDING THE ALKALINE DIET ... 12

What Does "Alkaline" Mean in Your Diet? ... 12

   Definition of pH and Its Importance ... 12

   How Foods Affect Body pH ... 13

   The pH Spectrum of Common Foods ... 15

Health Benefits of Alkaline Eating ... 18

   Potential Impact on Digestion and Metabolism ... 18

   Alkaline Diet and Chronic Disease Prevention ... 19

   Energy Levels and Mental Clarity ... 21

Dr. Sebi's Influence on Alkaline Eating ... 23

   Biography and Background of Dr. Sebi ... 23

   Key Components of Dr. Sebi's Diet ... 24

   Critiques and Scientific Perspective ... 25

CHAPTER 2: GETTING STARTED WITH YOUR ALKALINE TRANSITION ... 28

Preparing Your Kitchen for Alkaline Cooking ... 28

   Stocking Up on Alkaline Ingredients ... 28

   Organizing Your Space for Alkaline Cooking ... 29

Alkaline Substitutes for Everyday Ingredients ... 31

   Alternatives for Dairy, Gluten, and Refined Sugars ... 31

   Alkaline Spices and Seasonings ... 32

   Tips for Substituting Common Acidic Ingredients ... 34

RECIPES ... 36

Breakfast ... 36

   Avocado and Kale Smoothie ... 36

   Oat Flour Waffles ... 37

Pear and Amaranth Pudding	38
Kamut Toast with Spinach Pesto	39
Coconut Yogurt with Nuts and Berries	40
Spiced Teff Porridge	41
Blueberry Spelt Muffins	42
Buckwheat and Apricot Pancakes	43
Oatmeal Cream with Fresh Fruit and Nuts	44
Blueberry and Spinach Smoothie	45
Spelt Pancakes	46
Cinnamon Quinoa Porridge	47
Kamut Avocado Toast	48
Spelt Banana Muffins	49
Chia Berry Pudding	50
Tropical Smoothie	51
Alkaline Açaí Bowl	52
Seed and Nut Energy Bars	53
Chickpea Flour Vegan Omelette	54
Main Dishes	**55**
Farro Salad with Roasted Tomatoes	55
Beet and Ginger Soup	56
Chickpea Flour Crepes with Vegetables	57
Zucchini Spaghetti with Avocado Sauce	58
Quinoa with Asparagus and Toasted Almonds	59
Rice Pasta with Cilantro Pesto	60
Millet Risotto with Artichokes	61
Cucumber and Avocado Soup	62
Kamut Tagliatelle with Lemon and Thyme	63
Grilled Vegetable Quinoa Couscous with Tahini	64
Quinoa-Stuffed Bell Peppers with Sautéed Mushrooms and Zucchini	65
Zucchini Noodles with Avocado Pesto and Cherry Tomatoes	66
Butternut Squash and Lentil Curry	67
Spelt Flour Veggie Tacos	68
Baked Plantain and Sweet Potato Medley	69
Chickpea and Kale Stew	70

Spaghetti Squash with Alkaline Marinara Sauce	71
Portobello Mushroom Steaks with Garlic and Herbs	72
Alkaline Veggie Stir-Fry with Amaranth	73
Stuffed Eggplant with Millet and Herbs	74
Main Courses	75
Adzuki Bean and Sweet Potato Stew	75
Quinoa and Spinach Meatballs	76
Sesame Tofu and Broccoli	77
Green Curry Vegetables with Cauliflower Rice	78
Lentil and Squash Casserole	79
Vegetable Fajitas with Coconut Flour Tortillas	80
Portobello Mushroom and Quinoa Burger	81
Sweet and Sour Tempeh with Pineapple	82
Sweet Potato and Kale Gratin	83
Warm Chickpea and Roasted Vegetable Salad	84
Quinoa-Stuffed Bell Peppers with Alkaline Pesto	85
Butternut Squash and Lentil Curry	86
Spelt Pasta with Alkaline Alfredo Sauce	87
Grilled Vegetable Skewers with Spicy Tahini Sauce	88
Zucchini Noodles with Avocado Basil Sauce	89
Sides	90
Roasted Cauliflower with Paprika	90
Rosemary Roasted Potatoes	91
Avocado and Tomato Salad	92
Steamed Broccoli with Almond Sauce	93
Lemon and Mint Cucumber Salad	94
Grilled Zucchini with Basil	95
Carrot and Walnut Salad	96
Sautéed Spinach with Garlic and Lemon	97
Marinated Beetroot	98
Sautéed Asparagus and Mushrooms	99
Desserts	100
Mango Chia Seed Panna Cotta	100
Avocado and Chocolate Brownies	101

Lemon and Basil Sorbet	102
Alkaline Apple Cake	103
Lemon Poppy Seed Muffins	104
Almond and Ginger Cookies	105
Vanilla and Pecan Ice Cream	106
Peach and Raspberry Crumble	107
Date and Almond Bars	108
Pineapple and Coconut Cheesecake	109
Smoothie	110
Green Goddess Smoothie	110
Red Beet Reviver	111
Tropical Turmeric Cleanser	112
Berry Alkaline Boost	113
Minty Melon Mixer	114
Carrot Ginger Zing	115
Creamy Avocado Dream	116
Sweet Potato Pie Smoothie	117
Pineapple Parsley Punch	118
Spicy Cinnamon Apple Detox	119
QR-CODE MEAL PLAN	120

PREFACE

Introduction to the alkaline diet

Origins and Philosophy

The concept of the alkaline diet finds its roots in the early 20th century but gained significant prominence through the work of various natural health advocates. Among these, Dr. Sebi, a Honduran herbalist and self-proclaimed healer, stands out for his fervent promotion of alkaline foods as a pathway to health and vitality. The fundamental premise of the alkaline diet revolves around the idea that the foods we consume can directly influence the pH balance of our bodies, thereby affecting our overall health. Understanding the origins of the alkaline diet requires a brief dive into the history of pH science. The term "pH" stands for "potential of hydrogen" and is a measure of how acidic or alkaline a substance is, on a scale of 0 to 14. A pH of 7 is considered neutral, while values below 7 are acidic and above 7 are alkaline. Early research in the field of biochemistry suggested that maintaining a slightly alkaline pH in the blood is crucial for optimal health. This notion gave rise to the belief that diet could be manipulated to maintain this ideal pH balance.

Dr. Sebi, born Alfredo Bowman, became a pivotal figure in the promotion of the alkaline diet. His philosophy was heavily influenced by his own health challenges and his search for natural healing methods. After suffering from a range of ailments and finding no relief in conventional medicine, he turned to herbal medicine and dietary changes. His transformation led to the development of a unique dietary approach that emphasized the consumption of alkaline-rich foods, which he believed could detoxify the body, strengthen the immune system, and promote overall well-being.

Central to Dr. Sebi's philosophy was the idea that mucus is the root cause of disease. He posited that an acidic environment in the body leads to the production of excess mucus, which in turn clogs the system and creates a breeding ground for disease. By adopting an alkaline diet, he argued, one could reduce mucus production and thus eliminate the root cause of illness. This theory, though controversial and not widely accepted in the mainstream medical community, resonated with many people seeking alternative approaches to health. Dr. Sebi's diet is predominantly plant-based, focusing on natural, unprocessed foods that are believed to have alkalizing effects on the body. These include a variety of fruits, vegetables, nuts, and grains, with a strong emphasis on consuming foods that are as close to their natural state as possible. This approach aligns with the broader principles of natural hygiene and holistic health, which advocate for minimal intervention in the body's natural processes.

The alkaline diet also draws inspiration from traditional healing practices around the world. Many indigenous cultures have long recognized the importance of diet in maintaining health and preventing disease. For instance, Ayurvedic medicine from India and Traditional Chinese Medicine both emphasize the balance of different elements within the body, which includes maintaining an appropriate pH balance through dietary choices. These ancient practices have informed and enriched the modern understanding of the alkaline diet, providing a broader cultural and historical context for its principles. Critics of the alkaline diet often point out that the body has sophisticated mechanisms for regulating pH balance, primarily through the kidneys and lungs, which can effectively neutralize the impact of dietary acids and bases. However, proponents argue that while these mechanisms are indeed robust, they can be overwhelmed by a consistently acidic diet, leading to suboptimal health outcomes over time. This perspective underscores the importance of diet as a supportive factor in maintaining the body's natural balance.

The philosophy of the alkaline diet extends beyond mere pH balance; it encompasses a holistic approach to health that includes mental and emotional well-being. Dr. Sebi and other advocates often emphasize the importance of a positive mindset, stress reduction, and emotional resilience as integral components of a healthy lifestyle. This holistic view recognizes that physical health cannot be separated from mental and emotional health, and that achieving true wellness requires a comprehensive approach that addresses all aspects of the individual.

In essence, the origins and philosophy of the alkaline diet are deeply intertwined with a broader movement towards natural health and wellness. This movement challenges the conventional medical model, which often focuses on treating symptoms rather than addressing underlying causes. By advocating for a diet rich in alkaline foods, proponents of the alkaline diet aim to empower individuals to take control of their health through simple, natural, and accessible means. The enduring appeal of the alkaline diet lies in its promise of holistic health and its potential to offer a pathway to vitality and longevity. While scientific debate continues regarding the specifics of its mechanisms, the core principles of the alkaline diet—emphasizing natural, whole foods, and a balanced approach to health—resonate with a growing number of people seeking alternatives to conventional health practices. This blend of historical roots, cultural influences, and holistic philosophy forms the foundation of the alkaline diet and continues to inspire those who embrace its principles.

Core Principles of Alkaline Eating

Alkaline eating is more than a dietary preference; it's a holistic approach to nourishing the body, mind, and soul. At its heart lies a commitment to balance, purity, and natural living. These principles are designed to harmonize the body's internal environment, fostering optimal health and vitality. The core tenets of alkaline eating are grounded in the belief that the foods we consume have a profound impact on our body's pH levels, which in turn influences our overall well-being.

The first and perhaps most fundamental principle of alkaline eating is the emphasis on consuming whole, natural foods. This means prioritizing fruits, vegetables, nuts, seeds, and grains that are as close to their natural state as possible. Whole foods are rich in vitamins, minerals, and other essential nutrients that are vital for maintaining a healthy body. They are also free from the additives, preservatives, and other artificial ingredients commonly found in processed foods. By choosing whole foods, we align ourselves with the natural rhythms and cycles of the earth, fostering a deeper connection to the environment and our place within it. Another crucial principle is the importance of hydration. Water is essential for all bodily functions, from digestion and nutrient absorption to detoxification and temperature regulation. In the context of alkaline eating, hydration takes on an even greater significance. Alkaline advocates often emphasize the consumption of alkaline water, which has a higher pH than regular tap water. This type of water is believed to help neutralize acid in the bloodstream, support the body's natural detoxification processes, and promote better hydration at the cellular level. In addition to drinking plenty of water, consuming water-rich foods such as cucumbers, watermelon, and celery can further support optimal hydration and pH balance. The avoidance of acidic foods is another cornerstone of alkaline eating. Acidic foods, such as processed meats, dairy products, refined sugars, and artificial sweeteners, are thought to contribute to the body's acid load, leading to an imbalance in pH levels. Over time, a diet high in acidic foods can place a significant burden on the body's buffering systems, which work to maintain a stable pH in the blood and tissues. By minimizing the intake of these foods, we reduce the strain on these systems and allow the body to function more efficiently. This principle encourages mindful eating and a greater awareness of the types of foods we choose to nourish our bodies.

In tandem with avoiding acidic foods, alkaline eating promotes the consumption of alkaline-forming foods. These are foods that, once metabolized, contribute to a more alkaline environment in the body. Leafy green vegetables, such as kale, spinach, and Swiss chard, are excellent examples of alkaline-forming foods. They are rich in chlorophyll, vitamins, and minerals that support overall health and vitality. Other alkaline-forming foods include avocados, almonds, and certain grains like quinoa and amaranth. By incorporating a variety of these foods into our diet, we can help to balance our body's pH and support optimal health. A balanced approach to macronutrients is also central to alkaline eating. While many modern diets emphasize high protein or high-fat intake, the alkaline diet advocates for a more balanced distribution of carbohydrates, proteins, and fats. This balance is thought to support the body's natural functions and promote a more stable internal environment. Carbohydrates, particularly those from whole grains and vegetables, provide a steady source of energy, while healthy fats from sources like avocados, nuts, and seeds support cellular health and hormone production. Proteins, especially plant-based proteins from legumes and nuts, are essential for tissue repair and growth. By maintaining a balanced intake of these macronutrients, we can support overall health and well-being.

The principle of mindful eating is another key aspect of the alkaline diet. This involves being fully present during meals, savoring each bite, and paying attention to the body's hunger and satiety cues. Mindful eating encourages a deeper connection to the food we consume and promotes a greater appreciation for the nourishment it provides. It also helps to reduce overeating and supports better digestion and absorption of nutrients. By approaching meals with mindfulness, we can foster a more harmonious relationship with food and our bodies.

In addition to these dietary principles, alkaline eating also emphasizes the importance of lifestyle factors that support overall health. Regular physical activity, adequate sleep, and stress management are all considered vital components of an alkaline lifestyle. Exercise helps to improve circulation, support detoxification, and promote a healthy pH balance. Sleep is essential for the body's repair and regeneration processes, while stress management techniques such as meditation, deep breathing, and spending time in nature can help to reduce the body's acid load and promote a more alkaline state. By integrating these lifestyle practices with alkaline eating, we can create a holistic approach to health and well-being.

The principles of alkaline eating also extend to the way we source and prepare our food. Organic and sustainably grown foods are preferred, as they are free from harmful pesticides and chemicals that can contribute to the body's acid load. Cooking methods such as steaming, baking, and raw preparation are favored over frying or grilling, as they help to preserve the nutritional integrity of the foods. By choosing organic and sustainably sourced foods and using gentle cooking methods, we can further support our body's natural balance and promote optimal health. Ultimately, the core principles of alkaline eating are about more than just maintaining a certain pH level in the body. They reflect a broader commitment to living in harmony with the natural world, honoring the wisdom of our bodies, and making choices that support our overall well-being. By embracing these principles, we can create a foundation for a healthier, more vibrant life.

Common Misconceptions Clarified

The alkaline diet has garnered a significant following, but with its rise in popularity comes a host of misconceptions. Clarifying these misunderstandings is essential for anyone looking to adopt this lifestyle effectively. By dispelling myths, we can approach the alkaline diet with a clear and informed perspective, allowing its true benefits to shine through.

One of the most pervasive misconceptions is that the alkaline diet can change the pH of your blood. The human body is a complex system with stringent mechanisms to maintain a stable blood pH, usually around 7.4. This balance is tightly regulated by the kidneys and lungs, which work tirelessly to correct any deviations. While the foods you eat can influence the pH of your urine, they do not significantly alter the blood pH. This misunderstanding often leads to unrealistic expectations and can discourage individuals when they don't see immediate changes in their health metrics. Another common fallacy is that all acidic foods are unhealthy and should be entirely avoided. This is a simplistic view that overlooks the nutritional value of certain acidic foods. For instance, citrus fruits like lemons and oranges are acidic outside the body but have an alkalizing effect once metabolized. They are also rich in essential vitamins, antioxidants, and fiber. The key is not to eliminate all acidic foods but to maintain a balanced diet where alkaline-forming foods are predominant. There's also confusion around the term "alkaline-forming" foods. Many people assume that foods classified as alkaline-forming must taste bland or unappetizing. This is far from the truth. Alkaline-forming foods include a wide variety of delicious options such as avocados, almonds, quinoa, and a plethora of fruits and vegetables. By exploring these foods, one can discover new and exciting flavors while still adhering to the principles of alkaline eating.

The notion that the alkaline diet is overly restrictive is another misconception. While it does advocate for reducing the intake of processed and acidic foods, it also encourages a diverse and abundant consumption of whole, natural foods. This includes a broad spectrum of fruits, vegetables, grains, nuts, and seeds. The diet's emphasis is on inclusion rather than exclusion, promoting the idea of adding more nutrient-rich, alkaline-forming foods rather than focusing solely on what to cut out. This positive approach can lead to a more sustainable and enjoyable dietary practice.

Another myth is that the alkaline diet is scientifically unsupported. While it is true that some claims made by extreme proponents of the diet lack rigorous scientific backing, many aspects of the diet align with well-established nutritional principles. The emphasis on whole, plant-based foods, and the reduction of processed foods and sugars are recommendations that are widely supported by nutrition experts and health organizations. The confusion often arises from overreaching claims about the diet's ability to cure diseases or achieve unrealistic health outcomes.

Some critics argue that the alkaline diet is just another passing fad. However, its principles are rooted in long-standing dietary practices that emphasize natural, whole foods. These principles are not new; they echo traditional dietary guidelines from various cultures around the world that have been associated with longevity and good health. The alkaline diet's focus on balance and natural living can be seen as a return to these time-tested practices rather than a fleeting trend. A frequently encountered misconception is that the alkaline diet requires expensive, exotic foods that are difficult to find. While some specialized products may be marketed under the alkaline label, the core components of the diet are accessible and affordable. Staples such as leafy greens, root vegetables, whole grains, and nuts are readily available in most grocery stores. By prioritizing seasonal and locally grown produce, one can adhere to the alkaline diet without breaking the bank. There is also the belief that transitioning to an alkaline diet must be done all at once, which can be overwhelming for many people. In reality, adopting an alkaline diet can be a gradual process. Small, incremental changes, such as incorporating more vegetables into meals or replacing processed snacks with whole food alternatives, can lead to significant health benefits over time. This gradual approach makes the transition more manageable and sustainable.

Misunderstandings about the alkaline diet also extend to its perceived complexity. Some people think that following the diet requires extensive knowledge of food chemistry and constant monitoring of pH levels. While understanding the basics of how foods affect body pH is helpful, the diet itself can be quite straightforward. Focusing on a variety of whole, plant-based foods and listening to the body's signals can simplify the process. Overcomplicating the diet can create unnecessary stress and detract from its holistic and intuitive nature.

Lastly, there is the misconception that the alkaline diet is solely about diet and does not take into account other aspects of health. In truth, the alkaline philosophy encompasses a holistic approach to wellness. It recognizes the importance of physical activity, stress management, adequate sleep, and mental well-being as integral components of a healthy lifestyle. By considering these factors alongside dietary choices, individuals can achieve a more balanced and fulfilling state of health. Clarifying these common misconceptions helps to demystify the alkaline diet and allows individuals to make informed decisions about their health. By approaching the diet with a balanced and realistic perspective, one can appreciate its benefits without falling prey to unfounded myths. This clear understanding paves the way for a more successful and enjoyable experience with alkaline eating, fostering a deeper connection to one's health and well-being.

CHAPTER 1: UNDERSTANDING THE ALKALINE DIET

What Does "Alkaline" Mean in Your Diet?

Definition of pH and Its Importance

Understanding what "alkaline" means in your diet begins with grasping the concept of pH. The term pH stands for "potential of hydrogen" and Portions as a measure of how acidic or basic (alkaline) a substance is. This scale ranges from 0 to 14, where 7 is considered neutral. Numbers below 7 indicate acidity, while those above 7 denote alkalinity. The pH scale operates logarithmically, meaning each whole number represents a tenfold difference in hydrogen ion concentration. For example, a substance with a pH of 5 is ten times more acidic than one with a pH of 6. The importance of pH lies in its significant impact on various biochemical processes. For the human body, maintaining a stable pH, particularly in the blood, is critical for health. The optimal pH for human blood is tightly regulated around 7.4, slightly alkaline. Deviations from this range can disrupt cellular functions and metabolic processes, leading to health issues. The body's regulatory mechanisms, including the kidneys and lungs, work continuously to balance pH levels, underscoring the importance of pH to overall health.

Alkaline diets are based on the premise that consuming foods that promote a more alkaline internal environment can support these natural regulatory processes. This dietary approach emphasizes the intake of alkaline-forming foods, which are believed to help maintain or restore the body's optimal pH balance. Proponents of the alkaline diet argue that modern dietary patterns, which often include processed foods, refined sugars, and high protein intake, can lead to a more acidic internal environment, potentially compromising health over time. The historical context of pH and its relevance to health can be traced back to early studies in biochemistry. Researchers discovered that the body's pH balance plays a vital role in maintaining homeostasis, the state of steady internal conditions maintained by living organisms. Disruptions to this balance can affect enzyme function, oxygen transport, and overall metabolic efficiency. For example, an overly acidic environment can impair the function of enzymes, which are proteins that catalyze biochemical reactions essential for life. In addition to its biochemical importance, pH also influences the microbiome, the community of microorganisms living in the human gut. A balanced pH environment supports a healthy microbiome, which is crucial for digestion, nutrient absorption, and immune function. An acidic internal environment can disrupt this delicate balance, leading to dysbiosis, a condition characterized by an imbalance in the gut microbiota. Dysbiosis has been linked to various health issues, including digestive disorders, inflammation, and weakened immunity.

The alkaline diet's focus on promoting a more alkaline internal environment through dietary choices is thus rooted in a deep understanding of pH and its significance. By prioritizing alkaline-forming foods, individuals aim to support their body's natural pH regulatory mechanisms, potentially reducing the burden on these systems and promoting better health. This approach is not about radically altering the body's pH, which is not feasible through diet alone, but rather about supporting the body's existing efforts to maintain balance. Alkaline-forming foods typically include fruits, vegetables, nuts, and legumes, which are rich in vitamins, minerals, and antioxidants. These foods are contrasted with acid-forming foods, such as meat, dairy, processed foods, and refined sugars, which can contribute to an acidic internal environment when consumed in excess. The idea is to create a dietary pattern that leans towards alkalinity, supporting the body's natural pH balance and promoting overall health and well-being.

The concept of pH and its importance also extends to the broader environmental and lifestyle factors that can influence health. For instance, stress, lack of physical activity, and exposure to environmental toxins can all contribute to an acidic internal environment. The alkaline diet, therefore, often includes recommendations for holistic lifestyle changes that support pH balance, such as regular exercise, stress management techniques, and minimizing exposure to pollutants. Critics of the alkaline diet argue that the body is capable of maintaining pH balance regardless of dietary intake, thanks to its sophisticated regulatory mechanisms. While this is true to an extent, proponents of the diet contend that a supportive diet can ease the burden on these systems, particularly in the face of modern dietary and lifestyle challenges. The goal is not to override the body's natural functions but to assist them through mindful dietary choices. Understanding the definition of pH and its importance provides a foundational perspective for approaching the alkaline diet. It highlights the intricate balance the body maintains and underscores the potential benefits of dietary patterns that support this balance. While scientific debate continues regarding the extent of dietary impact on pH, the emphasis on whole, natural foods and a balanced approach to eating aligns with many established principles of good nutrition.

In essence, the pH scale is more than just a measure of acidity and alkalinity; it represents a critical aspect of human physiology and health. The alkaline diet's focus on pH underscores the broader goal of achieving and maintaining optimal health through natural, supportive means. By understanding and respecting the body's intricate balance, individuals can make informed choices that contribute to their overall well-being, rooted in the science of pH and its profound importance.

How Foods Affect Body pH

The concept of pH and its significance in human health is intricate, yet fascinating. To truly grasp how foods affect body pH, one must delve into the biochemical processes that occur post-consumption. The interaction between dietary choices and pH balance is a cornerstone of the alkaline diet, emphasizing the importance of selecting foods that promote an optimal internal environment.

When we consume food, it undergoes digestion, metabolism, and eventually, the residual ash–the end product of metabolic combustion–impacts the body's pH. This residual ash can be acidic, neutral, or alkaline, and it is this effect that influences the body's pH balance. It's crucial to understand that while the blood maintains a slightly alkaline pH around 7.4, the overall internal pH can fluctuate based on dietary inputs, albeit within a narrow range due to the body's regulatory mechanisms.

Proteins, primarily those from animal sources such as meat, fish, and dairy, tend to leave an acidic ash after metabolism. These foods contain high levels of sulfur-containing amino acids, phosphates, and other elements that metabolize into sulfuric and phosphoric acids. This acidic load can strain the body's buffering systems, which are designed to maintain pH homeostasis. The kidneys play a pivotal role in this process by excreting excess acids, but a prolonged high acid diet may contribute to a condition known as metabolic acidosis. This state is characterized by low-grade acidosis which can, over time, potentially lead to health issues such as kidney stones, osteoporosis, and muscle wasting.

Conversely, foods that are rich in potassium, magnesium, calcium, and other alkaline minerals generally produce an alkaline ash. Fruits and vegetables, for instance, are renowned for their alkalizing effects. These foods help neutralize excess acids in the body, supporting the kidneys and other buffering systems. For example, leafy greens, which are high in magnesium, play a significant role in maintaining muscle and nerve function while also contributing to the alkalizing effect. Similarly, bananas, which are rich in potassium, help in balancing the body's acid-base level.

The role of carbohydrates, particularly those derived from whole grains and legumes, is somewhat dualistic. While they are essential sources of energy, their effect on pH can vary. Whole grains such as quinoa and buckwheat tend to be more alkaline-forming, whereas refined grains can be more acid-forming due to their lack of essential nutrients and fiber. This demonstrates the importance of food quality and processing methods on their impact on body pH. Understanding the digestion process further elucidates how foods affect pH. For instance, the stomach's highly acidic environment (with a pH of around 2) is necessary for the initial breakdown of proteins. However, as the chyme (partially digested food) moves into the small intestine, the pancreas secretes bicarbonate to neutralize the acid, creating a more alkaline environment suitable for enzymatic activity. This shift illustrates the body's inherent ability to manage varying pH levels through complex biochemical pathways. Beyond macronutrients, micronutrients also play a crucial role in pH balance. Magnesium, calcium, and potassium are vital alkaline minerals that are abundant in many plant-based foods. These minerals not only aid in neutralizing acids but also support various physiological functions, including bone health, nerve transmission, and muscle function. For example, calcium from leafy greens and nuts helps buffer acid load and maintain bone density, illustrating the interplay between diet, mineral balance, and overall health.

Hydration also influences body pH. Water, particularly alkaline water, is thought to help neutralize acidity in the body. Hydration supports kidney function, which is essential for the excretion of excess acids. Adequate water intake ensures that the kidneys can effectively filter out toxins and maintain a balanced pH. This underscores the importance of not only what we eat but also what we drink in managing our internal pH environment. Stress and physical activity are additional factors that can affect body pH. High stress levels can lead to increased production of acid-forming hormones like cortisol. Physical activity, while beneficial for overall health, produces lactic acid during intense exercise. However, the overall benefits of regular physical activity outweigh the temporary production of lactic acid, as exercise also enhances the body's ability to manage and neutralize acid load through improved circulation and respiration. It's important to recognize that the body's buffering systems, including the kidneys, lungs, and bones, are incredibly efficient at maintaining pH balance. The lungs contribute by expelling carbon dioxide, a byproduct of metabolism that can form carbonic acid in the blood. Rapid or deep breathing can adjust pH by altering the level of carbon dioxide. The kidneys adjust the excretion of hydrogen ions and bicarbonate to balance pH. Bones act as a reservoir for calcium and other minerals that can be released to neutralize acids.

Despite the body's robust buffering capabilities, diet still plays a significant role in supporting these systems. By choosing foods that are predominantly alkaline-forming, we can reduce the strain on our buffering systems and promote overall health. This approach doesn't advocate for the complete elimination of acid-forming foods but rather encourages a balanced diet where alkaline-forming foods are more prominent.

In summary, the interaction between diet and body pH is a complex but critical aspect of health. By understanding how different foods affect pH, we can make informed dietary choices that support our body's natural regulatory mechanisms. This holistic approach not only fosters better health but also aligns with a broader commitment to natural and balanced living.

The pH Spectrum of Common Foods

The journey into understanding how the foods we consume affect our body's pH begins with a look at the pH spectrum of common foods. This spectrum ranges from highly acidic to highly alkaline, with each food leaving a residue, or "ash," that influences our internal pH balance once metabolized. Recognizing where foods fall on this spectrum is crucial for anyone looking to adopt an alkaline diet effectively. At the acidic end of the spectrum, we find foods that, despite their nutritional benefits, can contribute to an acidic internal environment. These include most animal proteins such as beef, pork, chicken, and fish. Dairy products like milk, cheese, and yogurt also fall into this category. When these foods are metabolized, they leave behind acidic byproducts such as phosphoric acid and sulfuric acid, which can lower the pH of the body's fluids. While these foods can be part of a balanced diet, their acidifying effects must be counterbalanced by alkaline-forming foods to maintain optimal pH levels. Processed foods and refined sugars are also highly acid-forming. Items such as white bread, pastries, candies, and soda contribute significantly to the body's acid load. These foods are typically low in essential nutrients and high in substances that metabolize into acids. Moreover, they can disrupt the balance of the gut microbiota, leading to further acid production and health issues such as inflammation and metabolic syndrome. Avoiding or minimizing these foods is a key principle of the alkaline diet, as their consumption can overwhelm the body's natural buffering systems.

Grains, particularly refined grains like white rice and pasta, also tend to be acid-forming. However, whole grains such as quinoa, brown rice, and millet are less acidic and provide essential nutrients and fiber, making them a better choice within the grain category. These whole grains, while still slightly acid-forming, are balanced by their nutritional benefits and should be consumed in moderation as part of a diverse diet.

On the neutral side of the spectrum, we have foods that neither significantly increase nor decrease the body's pH. These include certain fats and oils, like olive oil and avocados, as well as most legumes. Legumes, including lentils, chickpeas, and black beans, offer a substantial amount of protein and fiber without heavily influencing pH. They serve as excellent sources of plant-based nutrition and are pivotal in balancing the diet of those who follow an alkaline eating plan.

At the alkaline end of the spectrum, we encounter foods that help neutralize excess acids and promote a more alkaline internal environment. Leafy green vegetables, such as spinach, kale, and Swiss chard, are among the most alkaline-forming foods. They are rich in essential vitamins, minerals, and antioxidants that support overall health. These greens contribute significantly to alkalizing the body, aiding in the prevention of chronic diseases and promoting vitality.

Fruits, particularly those with low sugar content, also have alkaline-forming properties. Lemons, despite their acidic taste, are highly alkaline once metabolized, helping to balance the body's pH. Other fruits like watermelon, mangoes, and berries provide hydration and essential nutrients while promoting an alkaline environment. Their fiber content aids digestion and supports the gut microbiome, which plays a crucial role in maintaining pH balance.

Nuts and seeds, especially almonds and flaxseeds, are excellent alkaline-forming foods. They offer healthy fats, protein, and a variety of vitamins and minerals that support bodily functions and pH balance. Almonds, in particular, are noted for their high magnesium content, which plays a crucial role in numerous biochemical processes and helps maintain pH balance.

Root vegetables like sweet potatoes, carrots, and beets also contribute to alkalinity. These vegetables are not only nutrient-dense but also provide complex carbohydrates that sustain energy levels without causing significant acid formation. Their fiber content supports digestive health, further promoting an alkaline internal environment.

Herbs and spices, such as ginger, garlic, and turmeric, are noteworthy for their alkaline properties. These culinary additions enhance the flavor of dishes while providing anti-inflammatory and antioxidant benefits. They help to neutralize acids and support overall health, making them valuable components of an alkaline diet.

Hydration plays a vital role in maintaining pH balance, and water is the most neutral substance in terms of pH. Alkaline water, which has a higher pH than regular tap water, is believed to help neutralize acids in the body. While the science on alkaline water's benefits is still evolving, staying well-hydrated with clean, pure water supports the kidneys' role in pH regulation and overall health.

Fermented foods like sauerkraut, kimchi, and kefir, although slightly acidic due to their fermentation process, can be beneficial. They support a healthy gut microbiome, which is essential for maintaining pH balance and overall digestive health. The probiotics in fermented foods aid in the digestion of nutrients and help neutralize harmful acids in the gut.

Understanding the pH spectrum of common foods empowers individuals to make informed dietary choices that support their health goals. By incorporating more alkaline-forming foods and reducing the intake of acid-forming foods, one can help maintain a balanced internal environment. This approach aligns with the principles of the alkaline diet, emphasizing the importance of natural, whole foods and mindful eating practices. Navigating the pH spectrum of foods involves not just selecting the right ingredients but also considering preparation methods. Cooking techniques such as steaming, baking, and sautéing preserve the nutritional integrity of alkaline-forming foods, whereas frying or heavily processing foods can increase their acid-forming potential. Emphasizing gentle cooking methods helps retain the alkalizing benefits of foods and supports overall health. The interplay between diet and pH is complex, influenced by individual metabolic responses and overall lifestyle. While the pH spectrum provides a general guideline, personal experimentation and mindful eating are essential. Paying attention to how different foods affect one's body and making adjustments based on individual needs and responses can optimize health outcomes and promote a balanced internal environment.

In essence, the pH spectrum of common foods Portions as a foundational tool for those pursuing an alkaline diet. By understanding where foods fall on this spectrum and making conscious dietary choices, individuals can support their body's natural pH regulation, enhance overall well-being, and embrace a holistic approach to health.

Health Benefits of Alkaline Eating

Potential Impact on Digestion and Metabolism

The alkaline diet is often celebrated for its potential to improve digestion and metabolism, offering a pathway to better health and well-being. By focusing on foods that promote a more alkaline internal environment, this dietary approach can lead to significant benefits for the digestive system and metabolic processes.

Digestive health is foundational to overall well-being, and the alkaline diet supports this through its emphasis on natural, whole foods. Fruits, vegetables, nuts, and seeds, which are staples of this diet, are rich in dietary fiber. Fiber is crucial for healthy digestion as it adds bulk to the stool and facilitates regular bowel movements, preventing constipation and promoting a clean, efficient digestive tract. Moreover, fiber acts as a prebiotic, feeding the beneficial bacteria in the gut. A healthy gut microbiome is essential for efficient digestion and nutrient absorption, as well as for protecting against harmful pathogens.

Alkaline foods are also typically rich in water content, which aids in digestion. Proper hydration is necessary for the production of digestive enzymes and gastric juices that break down food. Hydrated foods like cucumbers, melons, and leafy greens support the body's ability to process and assimilate nutrients effectively. This hydration helps maintain the mucosal lining of the intestines, facilitating smooth and efficient digestion and reducing the risk of gastrointestinal discomfort. Furthermore, the alkaline diet encourages the reduction of acidic foods such as processed snacks, sugary drinks, and red meats, which can be harsh on the digestive system. These foods often lead to the overproduction of stomach acid, causing issues like acid reflux, heartburn, and indigestion. By minimizing these foods, the alkaline diet can help alleviate these common digestive complaints, promoting a more comfortable and efficient digestive process. Metabolism, the process by which the body converts food into energy, is another area where the alkaline diet shines. A diet rich in alkaline-forming foods can enhance metabolic efficiency by ensuring that the body operates in an optimal pH environment. Enzymatic reactions, which are crucial for metabolism, occur more efficiently in a slightly alkaline state. This means that the body can more effectively convert nutrients into energy, maintain healthy blood sugar levels, and regulate fat storage. Alkaline-forming foods, such as leafy greens, avocados, and nuts, provide essential nutrients that support metabolic health. Magnesium, found abundantly in spinach and almonds, plays a critical role in hundreds of enzymatic reactions, including those involved in energy production and glucose metabolism. Potassium, present in bananas and sweet potatoes, helps regulate fluid balance and muscle contractions, including those of the heart, which are vital for sustaining metabolic processes.

The alkaline diet's focus on reducing processed foods also helps stabilize blood sugar levels. Processed foods and refined sugars can cause spikes and crashes in blood glucose, leading to metabolic stress and increasing the risk of insulin resistance. By emphasizing whole foods with a low glycemic index, the alkaline diet promotes more stable blood sugar levels, enhancing metabolic function and reducing the risk of metabolic disorders like type 2 diabetes.

Additionally, an alkaline diet can aid in maintaining a healthy weight, which is closely linked to metabolic health. Alkaline foods are generally nutrient-dense yet lower in calories compared to processed and sugary foods. This combination of high nutrient density and lower calorie content can support weight management efforts, as it allows individuals to consume satisfying portions without excessive caloric intake. Maintaining a healthy weight reduces the strain on metabolic processes, making it easier for the body to sustain energy levels and overall health. Inflammation is another critical factor influenced by diet and metabolism. Acidic foods and high-sugar diets can contribute to chronic inflammation, which disrupts metabolic processes and leads to a host of health issues, including obesity, heart disease, and metabolic syndrome. The alkaline diet, rich in anti-inflammatory foods like leafy greens, berries, and nuts, helps combat inflammation. By reducing inflammation, the body can maintain more efficient metabolic processes and better overall health.

Furthermore, the alkaline diet supports the detoxification processes of the liver and kidneys, essential organs for metabolism. The liver plays a key role in metabolizing carbohydrates, fats, and proteins, and its efficient function is crucial for maintaining energy balance and metabolic health. By consuming foods that support liver health, such as cruciferous vegetables and citrus fruits, individuals can enhance the liver's ability to detoxify the body and regulate metabolism.

In summary, the alkaline diet's emphasis on whole, natural foods, hydration, and nutrient density offers a comprehensive approach to supporting digestive health and metabolic efficiency. By fostering a more alkaline internal environment, this dietary strategy can enhance enzymatic activity, stabilize blood sugar levels, reduce inflammation, and support the body's detoxification processes. This holistic approach not only improves digestion and metabolism but also contributes to overall health and vitality.

Alkaline Diet and Chronic Disease Prevention

Adopting an alkaline diet can be a powerful strategy in the prevention of chronic diseases, which are often linked to inflammation and oxidative stress in the body. The premise behind the alkaline diet is that by consuming alkaline-forming foods, you create a less hospitable environment for chronic diseases to develop and thrive. This approach is rooted in the idea that an alkaline internal environment can reduce inflammation, enhance cellular function, and support overall health, thereby mitigating the risk of chronic diseases.

Chronic diseases such as heart disease, diabetes, and certain cancers have been linked to dietary choices that promote an acidic environment in the body. Diets high in processed foods, refined sugars, and animal proteins can lead to an increase in acid load, which in turn can cause systemic inflammation. Inflammation is a key player in the development of many chronic diseases. By focusing on an alkaline diet, rich in fruits, vegetables, nuts, and seeds, individuals can significantly reduce their inflammatory markers.

Fruits and vegetables, which are staples of the alkaline diet, are rich in antioxidants and phytonutrients. These compounds help to neutralize free radicals, which are unstable molecules that can cause cellular damage and contribute to the development of chronic diseases. For instance, leafy greens like spinach and kale are packed with vitamins A, C, and E, all of which have potent antioxidant properties. These antioxidants help protect cells from damage, reduce inflammation, and improve overall immune function.

Moreover, the high fiber content of an alkaline diet plays a critical role in chronic disease prevention. Dietary fiber, abundant in fruits, vegetables, legumes, and whole grains, aids in the regulation of blood sugar levels and supports heart health by lowering cholesterol levels. Stable blood sugar levels are essential in preventing insulin resistance, a precursor to type 2 diabetes. Additionally, fiber promotes a healthy digestive system, which is crucial for the elimination of toxins and the maintenance of a balanced internal environment. The role of alkaline foods in supporting kidney function also cannot be understated. The kidneys are vital in maintaining acid-base balance in the body. Diets that are high in acid-forming foods can place a significant burden on the kidneys, leading to conditions such as kidney stones and chronic kidney disease. Alkaline-forming foods help to lighten this load, promoting better kidney function and reducing the risk of kidney-related issues. Citrus fruits, despite their acidic taste, are metabolized to produce alkaline byproducts that support renal health and overall detoxification processes. Bone health is another critical area where the alkaline diet offers significant benefits. Diets high in acidic foods can lead to the leaching of minerals from bones in an attempt to buffer excess acidity. This process can weaken bones and increase the risk of osteoporosis. Alkaline-forming foods, such as leafy greens and almonds, provide essential minerals like calcium and magnesium that are crucial for maintaining bone density and strength. By promoting a more alkaline internal environment, these foods help preserve bone health and reduce the risk of osteoporosis and fractures.

Cardiovascular health is deeply impacted by dietary choices, and the alkaline diet is no exception. Alkaline-forming foods are typically low in sodium and unhealthy fats, which are major contributors to high blood pressure and cardiovascular diseases. Instead, these foods are rich in potassium and healthy fats, which help regulate blood pressure and support heart health. Avocados, for example, are an excellent source of monounsaturated fats and potassium, both of which are beneficial for maintaining healthy blood pressure levels and reducing the risk of heart disease.

The connection between an alkaline diet and cancer prevention is also a subject of growing interest. While more research is needed to fully understand this relationship, some studies suggest that an alkaline environment can inhibit the growth of cancer cells. Cancer cells are known to thrive in acidic environments, and by reducing dietary acid load, it may be possible to create conditions that are less favorable for cancer development. Cruciferous vegetables like broccoli and Brussels sprouts, which are alkaline-forming, contain compounds that have been shown to have anti-cancer properties.

Mental health, though often overlooked in discussions about diet, is significantly influenced by what we eat. Chronic inflammation and oxidative stress are linked to mental health disorders such as depression and anxiety. The anti-inflammatory and antioxidant-rich foods that constitute the alkaline diet can help mitigate these effects, promoting better mental health and cognitive function. Omega-3 fatty acids, found in flaxseeds and walnuts, are particularly beneficial for brain health, reducing inflammation and supporting neuronal function.

In essence, the alkaline diet's emphasis on whole, natural foods supports the body's ability to maintain a balanced pH and reduces the risk factors associated with chronic diseases. By minimizing the intake of acid-forming foods and focusing on those that promote alkalinity, individuals can foster an internal environment conducive to long-term health and wellness. This holistic approach not only aids in the prevention of chronic diseases but also enhances overall quality of life by supporting the body's natural healing and maintenance processes.

Energy Levels and Mental Clarity

The alkaline diet is often praised not only for its physical health benefits but also for its positive effects on energy levels and mental clarity. By emphasizing nutrient-dense, natural foods, this dietary approach can significantly enhance overall vitality and cognitive function, leading to a more vibrant and focused life. A key factor in the relationship between the alkaline diet and energy levels is the reduction of systemic inflammation. Chronic inflammation, often fueled by diets high in processed foods, sugars, and unhealthy fats, can lead to fatigue and decreased energy levels. Alkaline-forming foods, such as fruits, vegetables, nuts, and seeds, are rich in antioxidants and anti-inflammatory compounds that help mitigate inflammation. This reduction in inflammation allows the body's systems to function more efficiently, conserving energy and promoting a sense of vitality.

Moreover, alkaline foods are typically abundant in essential vitamins and minerals that play crucial roles in energy production. Magnesium, found in leafy greens and nuts, is involved in over 300 enzymatic reactions, many of which are related to energy metabolism. Similarly, potassium, present in bananas and sweet potatoes, helps maintain proper cellular function and electrolyte balance, which are vital for sustaining energy levels throughout the day.

The alkaline diet also supports stable blood sugar levels, which are essential for maintaining consistent energy. Diets high in refined carbohydrates and sugars can lead to spikes and crashes in blood glucose, resulting in periods of hyperactivity followed by fatigue. Alkaline-forming foods, such as whole grains, legumes, and vegetables, have a low glycemic index, meaning they release glucose slowly into the bloodstream. This slow release prevents the sudden peaks and troughs associated with high-glycemic foods, promoting steady energy levels and reducing feelings of lethargy. Hydration is another critical aspect of the alkaline diet that contributes to energy and mental clarity. Proper hydration is essential for maintaining optimal physiological function, and many alkaline-forming foods are high in water content. Fruits like watermelon and cucumbers not only provide essential nutrients but also contribute to overall hydration. Adequate hydration ensures that the body's cells are functioning efficiently, which directly impacts energy levels. Dehydration, on the other hand, can lead to fatigue and impaired cognitive function.

Mental clarity, another significant benefit of the alkaline diet, is closely linked to the overall nutritional profile of the foods consumed. The brain requires a steady supply of nutrients to function optimally, and the alkaline diet provides these in abundance. Omega-3 fatty acids, found in flaxseeds and walnuts, are crucial for brain health. They support cognitive function, reduce inflammation in the brain, and improve communication between brain cells. These fats are essential for maintaining mental clarity and can help reduce symptoms of brain fog and cognitive decline. Antioxidants, prevalent in fruits and vegetables, also play a vital role in protecting the brain from oxidative stress. Oxidative stress occurs when there is an imbalance between free radicals and antioxidants in the body, leading to cellular damage. The antioxidants found in alkaline-forming foods neutralize free radicals, protecting brain cells from damage and supporting overall cognitive health. Blueberries, for example, are known for their high antioxidant content and have been linked to improved memory and cognitive function.

Additionally, the alkaline diet's emphasis on whole, unprocessed foods can lead to improved gut health, which is increasingly recognized as vital for mental clarity. The gut-brain axis, the communication network between the gastrointestinal tract and the brain, plays a crucial role in mental health. A healthy gut microbiome, supported by a diet rich in fiber and fermented foods, can improve mood, reduce anxiety, and enhance cognitive function. Fermented foods like sauerkraut and kimchi provide probiotics that support a healthy gut microbiome, which in turn positively impacts brain health. Stress management is another area where the alkaline diet can contribute to improved energy and mental clarity. Chronic stress can lead to adrenal fatigue, characterized by low energy levels and mental fog. Alkaline-forming foods help reduce stress levels by providing the nutrients necessary for adrenal health. Foods rich in vitamin C, such as bell peppers and citrus fruits, support adrenal function and help the body cope with stress more effectively.

Furthermore, the elimination of toxins through a diet rich in alkaline-forming foods can have profound effects on both energy levels and mental clarity. Processed foods often contain additives, preservatives, and other chemicals that can burden the liver and other detoxification organs. By reducing the intake of these substances and increasing the consumption of detoxifying foods like leafy greens and cruciferous vegetables, the body's detoxification pathways can function more efficiently. This detoxification process helps reduce the overall toxic load, resulting in clearer thinking and higher energy levels. In essence, the alkaline diet offers a holistic approach to improving energy levels and mental clarity. By focusing on nutrient-dense, anti-inflammatory, and hydrating foods, this diet supports the body's natural energy production processes and cognitive function. The result is not only a healthier body but also a sharper mind, capable of tackling daily challenges with greater vigor and focus. This holistic approach to diet and health underscores the profound connection between what we eat and how we feel, both physically and mentally.

Dr. Sebi's Influence on Alkaline Eating

Biography and Background of Dr. Sebi

Alfredo Darrington Bowman, better known as Dr. Sebi, was a Honduran herbalist and healer who became a prominent advocate for alkaline eating and natural health practices. Born on November 26, 1933, in Ilanga, Honduras, Dr. Sebi grew up in a rural environment, which profoundly influenced his approach to health and wellness. His early exposure to natural living and traditional healing methods set the stage for his later work in promoting alkaline diets and herbal medicine.

Dr. Sebi's journey into natural healing began with his own health struggles. In his thirties, he faced a myriad of health issues, including obesity, asthma, diabetes, and impotence. Conventional medical treatments failed to provide relief, prompting him to seek alternative approaches. His quest for healing led him to Mexico, where he met an herbalist who introduced him to the principles of herbal medicine and dietary changes. This encounter marked a turning point in Dr. Sebi's life, leading him to embrace a plant-based diet and natural remedies. Through this transformative experience, Dr. Sebi developed a deep understanding of the connection between diet and health. He became an ardent advocate for the consumption of natural, unprocessed foods and the avoidance of foods he believed to be detrimental to health, such as animal products, dairy, and refined sugars. Dr. Sebi's approach was rooted in the belief that an alkaline diet could detoxify the body, enhance vitality, and prevent disease. Dr. Sebi's philosophy was heavily influenced by his Afrocentric perspective, which emphasized the importance of returning to natural, indigenous practices for health and well-being. He believed that many of the health problems faced by people of African descent were due to the adoption of Western dietary habits, which he viewed as unnatural and harmful. By advocating for a diet based on alkaline foods and traditional herbs, Dr. Sebi sought to empower individuals to take control of their health through natural means.

In the 1980s, Dr. Sebi founded the USHA Research Institute in Honduras, named after his grandmother. The institute served as a center for natural healing and education, where Dr. Sebi and his team conducted research on the healing properties of various herbs and developed a range of herbal products. The institute also provided a sanctuary for individuals seeking to restore their health through natural methods, offering detoxification programs and dietary guidance. Dr. Sebi's work gained widespread attention in the 1980s when he claimed to have cured several individuals of serious diseases, including AIDS, cancer, and diabetes, using his herbal treatments and alkaline diet. These claims attracted both followers and skeptics, but they undeniably brought significant attention to his methods and philosophy. His bold statements and unconventional approach challenged the established medical community and sparked debates about the efficacy of natural healing. One of the most notable events in Dr. Sebi's career was his legal battle with the New York Attorney General's Office in 1988. He was charged with practicing medicine without a license and making false therapeutic claims. However, in a surprising turn of events, Dr. Sebi was acquitted after providing testimony from several patients who claimed to have been healed by his treatments. This legal victory bolstered his credibility and solidified his status as a pioneering figure in the field of natural health. Dr. Sebi's influence extended beyond his direct treatments and legal battles. He was also a prolific speaker and educator, sharing his knowledge through lectures, seminars, and written materials. His teachings emphasized the importance of an alkaline diet, regular detoxification, and the use of natural herbs to support the body's innate healing abilities. He encouraged individuals to question conventional medical practices and explore alternative approaches to health and wellness.

Throughout his life, Dr. Sebi remained dedicated to his mission of promoting natural health and empowering individuals to take control of their well-being. His work resonated with many people, particularly those disillusioned with conventional medicine and seeking holistic approaches to health. Dr. Sebi's legacy continues to inspire a growing movement of individuals committed to natural living and alkaline eating.

Dr. Sebi passed away on August 6, 2016, under circumstances that sparked controversy and speculation among his followers. Despite his death, his teachings and influence live on through the countless individuals who have embraced his principles and continue to advocate for natural health. His life's work remains a testament to the power of diet and natural remedies in promoting health and preventing disease. Dr. Sebi's impact on the field of natural health and alkaline eating is profound, and his legacy endures as a source of inspiration for those seeking alternative paths to wellness.

Key Components of Dr. Sebi's Diet

Dr. Sebi's diet, often referred to as the Dr. Sebi Nutritional Guide, is a distinctive approach to nutrition that emphasizes natural, plant-based foods believed to promote an alkaline internal environment. This dietary regimen is built on the premise that an alkaline body is less susceptible to disease and that consuming certain foods can help maintain this state. Dr. Sebi's diet is grounded in the idea of achieving optimal health through natural means, avoiding processed foods, and focusing on what he considered "electric" foods that support the body's bio-mineral balance.

Central to Dr. Sebi's diet is the exclusion of certain food groups that he believed contribute to the body's acidity and overall ill health. This includes the avoidance of all animal products such as meat, dairy, and eggs. Dr. Sebi argued that these foods are acid-forming and contribute to mucus buildup in the body, which he identified as a root cause of many diseases. By eliminating these foods, followers of his diet aim to reduce acidity and mucus production, thereby promoting better health. In addition to avoiding animal products, Dr. Sebi's diet strictly prohibits the consumption of processed and synthetic foods. This includes refined sugars, artificial sweeteners, preservatives, and food additives. Dr. Sebi believed that these substances disrupt the body's natural balance and lead to various health issues. Instead, his diet emphasizes whole, unprocessed foods that are as close to their natural state as possible. This approach is thought to enhance the body's ability to detoxify and maintain a healthy pH balance. One of the hallmark features of Dr. Sebi's diet is the focus on specific fruits and vegetables known for their alkalizing properties. Leafy greens like kale, spinach, and watercress are staples in his regimen due to their high chlorophyll content and mineral density. These vegetables are believed to help neutralize acids in the body and provide essential nutrients that support overall health. Other vegetables, such as cucumbers, zucchini, and bell peppers, are also encouraged for their hydrating and alkalizing effects.

Fruits play a significant role in Dr. Sebi's diet, particularly those with low sugar content. Berries, such as blueberries, raspberries, and strawberries, are favored for their antioxidant properties and alkalizing effects. Dr. Sebi also promoted the consumption of tropical fruits like mangoes, papayas, and soursop, which he believed offered unique health benefits and supported the body's natural detoxification processes. Another key component of Dr. Sebi's diet is the inclusion of certain grains and seeds that are considered alkaline-forming. Quinoa, amaranth, and wild rice are among the grains recommended for their nutrient density and ability to support digestive health. These grains provide essential amino acids, fiber, and minerals, contributing to a balanced and nutritious diet. Seeds like chia, flax, and hemp are also encouraged due to their healthy fat content and alkalizing properties.

Herbs and herbal teas are integral to Dr. Sebi's dietary approach. He identified specific herbs that he believed had powerful healing properties and could support the body's natural detoxification processes. Herbs such as burdock root, sarsaparilla, and dandelion are commonly used in his regimen to cleanse the blood, liver, and kidneys. These herbs are often consumed in tea form or as supplements, and they play a crucial role in maintaining the body's alkaline state.

Dr. Sebi's diet also emphasizes the importance of hydration with natural, spring water. He believed that proper hydration is essential for maintaining an alkaline environment and supporting the body's detoxification processes. Alkaline water, with its higher pH, is preferred as it is thought to help neutralize acids and promote overall health. Drinking plenty of water throughout the day is a key practice in Dr. Sebi's approach to health.

The concept of "electric" foods is a unique aspect of Dr. Sebi's diet. He used this term to describe foods that he believed were bio-electrically compatible with the human body, meaning they support the body's natural electrical activity and cellular function. According to Dr. Sebi, these foods help maintain the body's bio-mineral balance, promote optimal health, and prevent disease. Examples of "electric" foods include raw fruits and vegetables, nuts, seeds, and certain grains. Overall, Dr. Sebi's diet is a holistic approach to nutrition that prioritizes natural, plant-based foods while avoiding animal products, processed foods, and artificial substances. His emphasis on alkalizing foods, proper hydration, and the use of specific herbs reflects his belief in the body's innate ability to heal and maintain health when provided with the right nutrients. By adhering to these dietary principles, followers of Dr. Sebi's regimen aim to achieve a balanced internal environment, reduce the risk of disease, and enhance their overall well-being. This unique approach to eating has garnered a dedicated following and continues to influence those seeking alternative pathways to health.

Critiques and Scientific Perspective

Dr. Sebi's alkaline diet and his broader approach to natural healing have garnered both passionate support and considerable skepticism. To understand the full impact of his influence, it's essential to explore the critiques and scientific perspectives that surround his dietary principles and health claims.

One of the primary critiques of Dr. Sebi's approach is the lack of rigorous scientific evidence supporting his claims. While many followers report significant health improvements and even miraculous recoveries, these anecdotal accounts do not meet the stringent standards of scientific validation. The medical community generally requires large-scale, peer-reviewed studies to substantiate health claims, and such studies on Dr. Sebi's diet are notably absent. This gap in scientific literature leads to skepticism among healthcare professionals who emphasize evidence-based practice. Critics also point out that some of Dr. Sebi's dietary restrictions are extreme and may not be necessary for achieving health benefits. For instance, the complete avoidance of all animal products, processed foods, and hybrid plants is seen by some as overly restrictive and difficult to maintain. While there is consensus that reducing processed foods and increasing the intake of fruits and vegetables is beneficial, the total exclusion of certain food groups without individualized dietary assessment can potentially lead to nutritional deficiencies if not properly managed. The scientific perspective on the body's pH balance also diverges from Dr. Sebi's teachings. The body regulates its pH levels through complex homeostatic mechanisms involving the lungs and kidneys, which maintain a blood pH around 7.4. Critics argue that dietary choices have a limited impact on blood pH due to these regulatory systems. They contend that while diet can influence the pH of urine, this is not indicative of systemic changes in the body's overall pH balance. Thus, the notion that an alkaline diet can significantly alter blood pH and prevent disease is viewed with skepticism by many in the medical field.

Additionally, the concept of "mucus" as a root cause of disease, central to Dr. Sebi's philosophy, lacks scientific support. Modern medicine recognizes that mucus production is a natural and protective response of the body, playing crucial roles in respiratory and digestive health. While excessive mucus production can be symptomatic of underlying health issues, it is not widely accepted as the primary cause of disease. This fundamental difference in understanding contributes to the divide between Dr. Sebi's followers and the scientific community. Despite these critiques, there are aspects of Dr. Sebi's diet that align with established nutritional principles. The emphasis on plant-based foods, for instance, is consistent with a wealth of research supporting the health benefits of diets rich in fruits, vegetables, nuts, and seeds. These foods are known for their anti-inflammatory properties, high nutrient density, and positive effects on chronic disease prevention. In this regard, Dr. Sebi's diet echoes recommendations from various health organizations advocating for increased consumption of whole, plant-based foods.

Moreover, the holistic approach of Dr. Sebi's diet, which considers overall lifestyle factors such as stress reduction, hydration, and natural living, resonates with contemporary movements towards integrative health. There is growing recognition of the importance of lifestyle and dietary patterns in maintaining health and preventing disease. This broader perspective, which includes dietary practices as one component of overall well-being, reflects an understanding that health is multifaceted and influenced by a combination of factors.

Some scientific studies indirectly support elements of Dr. Sebi's diet, particularly the benefits of specific plant-based foods and herbs. For example, research on the anti-inflammatory and antioxidant properties of various fruits and vegetables aligns with Dr. Sebi's recommendations. Herbs such as burdock root and dandelion, which are part of his dietary regimen, have been studied for their potential health benefits, including detoxification and anti-inflammatory effects. While these studies do not specifically validate Dr. Sebi's entire approach, they do lend credence to some of the individual components of his diet. The critiques and scientific perspectives on Dr. Sebi's influence highlight a broader discussion about the role of alternative medicine and holistic health approaches in contemporary healthcare. While there is skepticism and a need for more rigorous research, the popularity and reported benefits of Dr. Sebi's diet suggest that many individuals find value in his teachings. This underscores the importance of ongoing dialogue between conventional medicine and alternative health practices to explore potential integrative approaches that can benefit patients.

In summary, Dr. Sebi's influence on alkaline eating is marked by both passionate advocacy and critical scrutiny. While his claims and dietary principles challenge conventional scientific understanding, they also resonate with a significant number of people seeking natural and holistic approaches to health. The intersection of critique and support reflects the complexities of integrating traditional and alternative health practices, highlighting the need for further research and open-minded exploration of diverse approaches to wellness.

CHAPTER 2: GETTING STARTED WITH YOUR ALKALINE TRANSITION

Preparing Your Kitchen for Alkaline Cooking

Stocking Up on Alkaline Ingredients

Creating an alkaline kitchen starts with understanding which ingredients support an alkaline diet and then stocking up on those essentials. This process transforms your kitchen into a haven for healthy, vibrant eating and ensures that you have the right tools at your fingertips to prepare nourishing meals that promote optimal health.

The foundation of an alkaline diet is built on a variety of fresh, whole foods that help maintain the body's pH balance. Fresh fruits and vegetables are at the core of this dietary approach. Leafy greens such as kale, spinach, and Swiss chard are particularly alkaline and rich in essential nutrients like magnesium, calcium, and vitamins A, C, and K. These greens can be used in salads, smoothies, and stir-fries, providing versatility in your daily meal preparation. Cruciferous vegetables such as broccoli, cauliflower, and Brussels sprouts are also key players in an alkaline kitchen. These vegetables are known for their detoxifying properties and high fiber content, which support digestion and overall health. Including a variety of these vegetables in your diet ensures a broad spectrum of nutrients and flavors. Fruits, while sometimes debated due to their natural sugar content, are an important part of the alkaline diet when chosen wisely. Berries, such as blueberries, strawberries, and raspberries, are excellent choices due to their high antioxidant content and lower glycemic index. Citrus fruits like lemons and limes, despite their acidic taste, have an alkalizing effect on the body once metabolized and can be used to add flavor to water, salads, and marinades. Hydration is crucial in an alkaline diet, so stocking up on ingredients that support this is essential. Cucumber and watermelon are highly alkaline and hydrating, making them perfect additions to salads, smoothies, or simply enjoyed on their own. Coconut water is another excellent hydrating option that provides electrolytes and aids in maintaining an alkaline state.

Nuts and seeds, though calorie-dense, offer healthy fats and proteins that are important in an alkaline diet. Almonds and flaxseeds are particularly beneficial due to their omega-3 fatty acid content, which has anti-inflammatory properties. These can be added to smoothies, oatmeal, or enjoyed as a snack to provide a nutritious and satisfying option.

Whole grains and legumes also play a vital role in an alkaline diet. Quinoa, amaranth, and millet are alkaline-forming grains that offer essential amino acids, fiber, and minerals. They can serve as a base for meals, providing a satisfying and nutrient-dense option. Legumes, such as lentils and chickpeas, are not only alkaline but also high in protein and fiber, making them a staple in an alkaline kitchen.

Herbs and spices are not only flavorful additions to meals but also contribute to the alkalinity of the diet. Fresh herbs like basil, cilantro, and parsley are highly alkaline and can be used to enhance the flavor of dishes while providing additional health benefits. Spices such as turmeric and ginger have anti-inflammatory properties and can be incorporated into teas, soups, and main dishes to boost both flavor and nutrition.

Healthy oils are another crucial component of an alkaline kitchen. Olive oil and coconut oil are preferred choices due to their health benefits and versatility in cooking. These oils can be used in salad dressings, for sautéing vegetables, or in baking, adding healthy fats to your diet without compromising alkalinity.

Proper storage of these ingredients is vital to maintain their freshness and nutritional value. Fresh produce should be stored in a way that maximizes its shelf life, such as keeping leafy greens and herbs in the refrigerator in perforated bags to allow for air circulation. Nuts and seeds should be stored in airtight containers to prevent them from going rancid, and whole grains and legumes should be kept in cool, dry places to maintain their quality.

Building an alkaline pantry also involves incorporating natural sweeteners and avoiding refined sugars. Options like raw honey, maple syrup, and stevia provide sweetness without the acid-forming properties of processed sugars. These can be used in baking, beverages, and as toppings for various dishes. Transitioning to an alkaline kitchen may require some initial investment and adjustment, but the benefits of having a well-stocked pantry with alkaline ingredients are substantial. It enables the preparation of meals that are not only delicious but also support the body's natural balance and overall health. By focusing on fresh, whole foods and avoiding processed ingredients, you create an environment that promotes wellness and vitality, making the journey towards an alkaline diet both practical and enjoyable.

Organizing Your Space for Alkaline Cooking

Creating a kitchen environment conducive to alkaline cooking involves thoughtful organization and strategic placement of tools and ingredients. This ensures that your kitchen is not only efficient but also inspiring, making it easier to maintain a healthy and balanced diet. Proper organization can transform your cooking space into a sanctuary for preparing nourishing meals that support an alkaline lifestyle.

Start by evaluating your kitchen layout and storage options. A well-organized kitchen begins with decluttering. Remove items that you no longer use or that do not align with your alkaline eating goals. This creates space for the essential tools and ingredients that will become the foundation of your new cooking habits. Consider donating or repurposing old kitchen gadgets and non-alkaline pantry items to make room for healthier alternatives. Next, prioritize accessibility. The items you use most frequently should be easily reachable. Store fresh produce, nuts, seeds, and other staples in clear containers within easy reach. This not only keeps them fresh but also Portions as a visual reminder of your commitment to an alkaline diet. Clear containers help you see what you have at a glance, reducing food waste and ensuring you always have essential ingredients on hand. Arrange your pantry in a way that groups similar items together. Place grains like quinoa, amaranth, and millet in one section, while keeping legumes such as lentils and chickpeas in another. This organization helps streamline meal preparation, allowing you to quickly locate what you need. Labeling containers can further enhance this system, making it simple to identify ingredients and manage your inventory.

The refrigerator should also be organized to support alkaline cooking. Store leafy greens, vegetables, and fruits in designated areas, preferably in the crisper drawers to maintain their freshness. Use separate containers for different types of produce to prevent cross-contamination and extend their shelf life. Storing herbs in a glass of water in the refrigerator can keep them fresh for longer, ready to add flavor and nutrients to your meals. Dedicate a section of your kitchen to herbs and spices. These are crucial for adding flavor and nutritional value to your dishes. Store herbs and spices in a cool, dry place away from direct sunlight. Consider using a spice rack or drawer organizer to keep them neatly arranged and easily accessible. This setup not only keeps your kitchen tidy but also encourages you to experiment with different flavors, making your meals more enjoyable. Cooking utensils and equipment should be organized based on their frequency of use. Essential tools for alkaline cooking, such as a high-quality blender for smoothies, a food processor for chopping vegetables, and a juicer for fresh juices, should be kept on the countertop or in easily accessible cabinets. Less frequently used items can be stored in higher or lower cabinets, freeing up prime space for daily essentials. Incorporate sustainable and eco-friendly storage solutions wherever possible. Glass containers, reusable silicone bags, and beeswax wraps are excellent alternatives to plastic and can help keep your ingredients fresh without contributing to environmental waste. These sustainable options are not only better for the planet but also align with the holistic approach of the alkaline diet. Creating a designated prep area is another key aspect of organizing your kitchen for alkaline cooking. This space should be equipped with a cutting board, sharp knives, and other essential tools. Keeping this area clean and clutter-free makes it easier to prepare meals efficiently and reduces stress during cooking. Consider adding a compost bin nearby to dispose of vegetable scraps, promoting a more sustainable kitchen environment.

Meal planning and preparation can be greatly enhanced by organizing your kitchen. Keep a whiteboard or notepad in your kitchen to jot down grocery lists, meal ideas, and reminders. This practice helps ensure that you always have the necessary ingredients for your planned meals and reduces the temptation to rely on convenience foods that may not align with your dietary goals.

Incorporate elements that inspire and motivate you to maintain an alkaline lifestyle. This could include displaying cookbooks with alkaline recipes, hanging inspirational quotes, or keeping a fruit bowl on the counter as a visual reminder of your commitment to healthy eating. Surrounding yourself with positive cues can reinforce your goals and make your kitchen a place of joy and creativity.

Finally, regular maintenance is key to keeping your kitchen organized and efficient. Set aside time each week to tidy up, check your inventory, and plan your meals. This habit ensures that your kitchen remains a supportive environment for alkaline cooking and that you are always prepared to create nutritious and delicious meals. By thoughtfully organizing your kitchen space, you can create an environment that supports and enhances your alkaline cooking journey. An efficient, well-arranged kitchen not only makes meal preparation easier but also reinforces your commitment to a healthy lifestyle. With the right setup, your kitchen can become a hub of nourishment and well-being, helping you achieve and maintain your health goals.

Alkaline Substitutes for Everyday Ingredients

Alternatives for Dairy, Gluten, and Refined Sugars

Transitioning to an alkaline diet often involves replacing common acidic ingredients with healthier, alkaline alternatives. This process can seem daunting at first, but with the right knowledge and substitutions, you can enjoy delicious, nourishing meals that support your health goals. Here, we'll explore effective alternatives for dairy, gluten, and refined sugars, providing you with the tools to make seamless swaps in your everyday cooking. Dairy products are a staple in many diets, but they can be highly acidic and contribute to mucus production and inflammation. Fortunately, there are several alkaline-friendly substitutes that can replace dairy in most recipes without sacrificing taste or texture. Almond milk, for example, is an excellent substitute for cow's milk. It has a mild flavor that works well in both sweet and savory dishes. Rich in vitamin E and healthy fats, almond milk can be used in smoothies, baking, and even in your morning coffee.

Coconut milk is another versatile option, especially for cooking and baking. It adds a creamy texture and subtle sweetness to dishes, making it perfect for soups, curries, and desserts. Coconut milk is also packed with medium-chain triglycerides (MCTs), which provide a quick source of energy and support metabolic health. For those who prefer a nut-free option, oat milk is a great choice. It has a naturally sweet taste and works well in baking, as well as in beverages like lattes and smoothies.

Cheese, another beloved dairy product, can also be replaced with alkaline alternatives. Nutritional yeast, for instance, offers a cheesy flavor without the acidity of dairy. It is high in B vitamins and can be sprinkled on popcorn, pasta, and salads. Cashew cheese is another delicious substitute that can be made at home by blending soaked cashews with lemon juice, nutritional yeast, and seasonings. It's creamy, tangy, and can be used in a variety of dishes, from dips to spreads to sauces.

Gluten, found in wheat, barley, and rye, is another common ingredient that many people seek to avoid due to its potential inflammatory effects and difficulty in digestion. Fortunately, there are numerous gluten-free grains and flours that are more alkaline and can easily replace traditional wheat products. Quinoa, for example, is a highly nutritious grain that is naturally gluten-free and alkaline. It can be used as a base for salads, in soups, or as a side dish. Quinoa flour is also available and can be used in baking.

Amaranth and millet are other excellent gluten-free grains that are alkaline and rich in nutrients. They can be cooked similarly to rice and used in a variety of dishes. For baking, almond flour and coconut flour are popular choices. Almond flour is made from finely ground almonds and adds a rich, nutty flavor to baked goods. Coconut flour, made from dried coconut meat, is highly absorbent and best used in combination with other flours. Both of these flours are excellent for making breads, muffins, and pancakes.

Refined sugars are highly acidic and contribute to a host of health issues, including inflammation, weight gain, and blood sugar imbalances. Replacing refined sugars with more natural, alkaline options is a key step in maintaining an alkaline diet. Stevia, a natural sweetener derived from the leaves of the stevia plant, is a zero-calorie alternative that does not spike blood sugar levels. It can be used in beverages, baking, and cooking.

Maple syrup and raw honey are other great substitutes for refined sugars. While they are sweeter than stevia and contain some natural sugars, they also offer additional nutrients. Maple syrup contains minerals such as zinc and manganese, while raw honey has antibacterial properties and is rich in antioxidants. These natural sweeteners can be used in moderation to sweeten desserts, dressings, and beverages.

Dates and date syrup provide another excellent alternative to refined sugar. Dates are naturally sweet and packed with fiber, vitamins, and minerals. Blending dates into smoothies, using date syrup in baking, or incorporating them into sauces can provide sweetness along with nutritional benefits. Similarly, coconut sugar, made from the sap of coconut palms, is a less processed sweetener that retains some nutrients and has a lower glycemic index than refined sugar.

Making these substitutions may require some experimentation to get the flavors and textures just right, but the benefits are well worth the effort. By replacing acidic ingredients with these healthier, alkaline alternatives, you can create meals that are not only delicious but also supportive of your overall health. Whether you're making a creamy sauce, baking bread, or sweetening your tea, these swaps will help you maintain an alkaline diet and enjoy a wide variety of satisfying foods.

Alkaline Spices and Seasonings

Enhancing the flavor of your meals while adhering to an alkaline diet is not only possible but can also be an exciting culinary adventure. Alkaline spices and seasonings add depth, complexity, and nutritional benefits to your dishes without compromising the principles of alkaline eating. Understanding which spices and seasonings are alkaline-friendly and how to use them effectively can transform your cooking and support your health goals.

Herbs and spices are the cornerstone of any flavorful dish, and many of them are highly alkaline and packed with beneficial compounds. Fresh herbs like basil, cilantro, and parsley are excellent choices. Basil, with its sweet and slightly peppery flavor, is a versatile herb that can be used in salads, pesto, and as a garnish for a variety of dishes. It's rich in antioxidants and has anti-inflammatory properties. Cilantro, known for its distinct, refreshing taste, is often used in salsas, salads, and as a topping for soups and tacos. It helps detoxify heavy metals from the body and supports digestive health. Parsley, with its mild, slightly bitter flavor, is commonly used as a garnish but can also be added to smoothies, salads, and sauces for a nutrient boost. It's high in vitamins A, C, and K, and supports kidney function.

Spices also play a crucial role in an alkaline diet. Turmeric, a golden-yellow spice commonly used in Indian cuisine, is renowned for its anti-inflammatory and antioxidant properties. It contains curcumin, which has been shown to reduce inflammation and improve brain function. Turmeric can be used in soups, stews, curries, and even smoothies. Combining turmeric with black pepper enhances its bioavailability, making it more effective.

Ginger, another powerful spice, adds a warm, slightly spicy flavor to dishes and has numerous health benefits. It aids digestion, reduces nausea, and has anti-inflammatory effects. Fresh ginger can be grated into teas, smoothies, and stir-fries, while powdered ginger is perfect for baking and spice blends. Garlic, known for its pungent flavor, is a staple in many cuisines and offers significant health benefits, including boosting the immune system and reducing blood pressure. Fresh garlic can be used in virtually any savory dish, from soups and sauces to roasted vegetables and dressings.

Cayenne pepper, with its fiery heat, is an excellent way to add spice to your meals while reaping health benefits. It contains capsaicin, which boosts metabolism, reduces hunger, and has pain-relieving properties. Cayenne can be added to soups, stews, and even detox drinks for a spicy kick.

Other alkaline spices include cinnamon and cumin. Cinnamon, known for its sweet and warm flavor, can help regulate blood sugar levels and is high in antioxidants. It's perfect for adding to smoothies, oatmeal, and baked goods. Cumin, with its earthy and slightly spicy flavor, aids digestion and is rich in iron. It's commonly used in spice blends, curries, and roasted vegetables. Incorporating these spices into your meals can enhance flavor and provide numerous health benefits. For instance, creating spice blends allows you to combine multiple alkaline spices into a convenient seasoning mix. A homemade curry powder blend might include turmeric, cumin, coriander, ginger, and black pepper, providing a balanced and flavorful addition to any dish. Similarly, a taco seasoning blend with cumin, paprika, garlic powder, and cayenne pepper can be used to season vegetables, beans, and grains. Fresh herbs can also be transformed into sauces and dressings. A basil pesto made with fresh basil, garlic, olive oil, and nuts is a versatile sauce that can be used on pasta, sandwiches, and as a dip for vegetables. A cilantro-lime dressing can be made by blending fresh cilantro, lime juice, olive oil, and a touch of honey, perfect for salads and grain bowls. Dried herbs and spices should be stored properly to maintain their potency and flavor. Keeping them in airtight containers away from light and heat will ensure they remain fresh and effective. Regularly refreshing your spice collection also helps to keep your cooking vibrant and flavorful.

Exploring different cuisines is another way to incorporate a variety of alkaline spices and seasonings into your diet. Middle Eastern, Indian, and Mediterranean cuisines, for example, make extensive use of alkaline-friendly spices and herbs. Trying recipes from these culinary traditions can introduce you to new flavors and cooking techniques, keeping your meals exciting and varied. Ultimately, the key to successfully using alkaline spices and seasonings is to experiment and find combinations that you enjoy. By doing so, you not only enhance the flavor of your meals but also boost their nutritional profile, supporting your journey towards better health and wellness. Embracing the rich array of alkaline spices and seasonings available can make your culinary experience both delicious and healthful.

Tips for Substituting Common Acidic Ingredients

Transforming your kitchen into an alkaline-friendly space involves making thoughtful substitutions for common acidic ingredients. By choosing alternatives that support an alkaline diet, you can maintain the flavors and textures you love while promoting better health. Here are some practical tips for substituting common acidic ingredients with alkaline-friendly options.

Traditional flour is a staple in many recipes but is highly acidic and often gluten-containing. Almond flour and coconut flour are excellent alkaline substitutes. Almond flour, made from finely ground almonds, provides a rich, nutty flavor and is perfect for baking cakes, muffins, and bread. Coconut flour, on the other hand, is highly absorbent and works well in combination with other flours. It adds a subtle sweetness and is ideal for making pancakes and cookies. For those seeking a more neutral flavor, quinoa flour and amaranth flour are great choices. They can be used in baking and cooking to create a variety of dishes without compromising on taste or nutritional value.

Refined sugars are another common acidic ingredient that can be replaced with alkaline-friendly sweeteners. Stevia, derived from the leaves of the stevia plant, is a natural, zero-calorie sweetener that can be used in beverages, desserts, and baking. It is significantly sweeter than sugar, so a small amount goes a long way. Maple syrup and raw honey are also excellent substitutes, offering a rich flavor and additional nutrients. Maple syrup contains minerals like zinc and manganese, while raw honey provides antioxidants and has antibacterial properties. These sweeteners can be used in moderation to enhance the flavor of your recipes.

Milk and cream, staples in many households, can be substituted with various plant-based milks. Almond milk and coconut milk are popular choices due to their mild flavors and versatility. Almond milk is great for smoothies, cereals, and baking, while coconut milk adds a creamy texture to soups, curries, and desserts. Oat milk, another excellent option, is naturally sweet and works well in coffee, lattes, and baked goods. For a richer alternative, cashew milk can be used, offering a creamy consistency ideal for sauces and ice creams.

Cheese, a beloved ingredient in many dishes, can be replaced with nutritional yeast and cashew-based cheeses. Nutritional yeast has a cheesy, nutty flavor and is packed with B vitamins. It can be sprinkled on popcorn, pasta, and salads. Cashew cheese, made by blending soaked cashews with lemon juice, nutritional yeast, and seasonings, is a versatile alternative that can be used as a dip, spread, or in sauces. This creamy, tangy substitute is perfect for those looking to reduce their intake of dairy while enjoying the rich flavors of traditional cheese.

Eggs, commonly used in baking and cooking, can be substituted with several alkaline-friendly options. For baking, flaxseeds or chia seeds mixed with water create a gel-like consistency that mimics the binding properties of eggs. One tablespoon of ground flaxseeds or chia seeds mixed with three tablespoons of water can replace one egg in most recipes. For savory dishes, mashed bananas or applesauce can be used as egg substitutes, adding moisture and a slight sweetness to the final product. Silken tofu, blended until smooth, is another excellent egg substitute for baking and cooking, providing a similar texture without the acidity of eggs.

Butter and other oils can be substituted with healthier, alkaline-friendly fats. Coconut oil and olive oil are both excellent choices. Coconut oil, with its mild coconut flavor, is great for baking, sautéing, and frying. Olive oil, known for its heart-healthy benefits, can be used in dressings, marinades, and for light sautéing. Avocado oil is another versatile option, offering a neutral flavor and high smoke point, making it suitable for cooking and baking.

Soy sauce, a common seasoning in many dishes, is acidic and can be replaced with tamari or coconut aminos. Tamari is a gluten-free soy sauce alternative that provides a similar umami flavor without the acidity. Coconut aminos, made from fermented coconut sap, offer a slightly sweeter and less salty flavor compared to soy sauce. They can be used in stir-fries, marinades, and as a dipping sauce, providing a flavorful alternative that supports an alkaline diet.

White vinegar, often used in dressings and marinades, is acidic and can be replaced with apple cider vinegar or lemon juice. Apple cider vinegar, made from fermented apples, offers a milder acidity and additional health benefits, such as aiding digestion and balancing blood sugar levels. Lemon juice, with its fresh, tangy flavor, is another excellent substitute that adds brightness to salads, sauces, and marinades.

Incorporating these alkaline substitutes into your cooking and baking not only supports your health but also opens up a world of new flavors and textures. By making these simple swaps, you can enjoy a variety of delicious, nourishing meals that align with your alkaline eating goals. Experimenting with these alternatives can transform your kitchen into a hub of creativity and wellness, ensuring that every meal is both satisfying and beneficial.

RECIPES

Breakfast

Avocado and Kale Smoothie

Portions: 2

Ingredients:

- 1 ripe avocado
- 2 cups kale leaves, chopped
- 1 banana
- 1 cup almond milk
- 1 tablespoon chia seeds
- 1 tablespoon honey (optional)
- Ice cubes

Preparation Time: 10 minutes

Nutritional Information (per serving):

Calories	Carbohydrates	Protein	Fat	Fiber	Sugar
220 kcal	28 g	4 g	12 g	9 g	14 g

Instructions:

1. Cut the avocado in half, remove the pit, and scoop out the flesh.
2. In a blender, combine the avocado, kale, banana, almond milk, chia seeds, and honey (if using).
3. Blend until smooth. If the smoothie is too thick, add more almond milk or water to achieve the desired consistency.
4. Add ice cubes and blend again until the ice is crushed and well mixed.
5. Pour into glasses and serve immediately.

Tips:

- For added protein, you can include a scoop of protein powder.
- Use frozen banana slices for a thicker, colder smoothie.

Oat Flour Waffles

Portions: 4

Ingredients:

- 2 cups oat flour
- 2 tablespoons sugar
- 1 tablespoon baking powder
- 1/2 teaspoon salt
- 2 large eggs
- 1 1/2 cups milk (dairy or non-dairy)
- 1/4 cup melted coconut oil
- 1 teaspoon vanilla extract

Preparation Time: 20 minutes

Nutritional Information (per serving):

Calories	Carbohydrates	Protein	Fat	Fiber	Sugar
320 kcal	45 g	8 g	12 g	6 g	8 g

Instructions:

1. Preheat your waffle iron.
2. In a large bowl, whisk together the oat flour, sugar, baking powder, and salt.
3. In another bowl, beat the eggs and then add the milk, melted coconut oil, and vanilla extract.
4. Pour the wet ingredients into the dry ingredients and stir until just combined.
5. Lightly grease the waffle iron with cooking spray or a little coconut oil.
6. Pour enough batter into the waffle iron to cover the surface (amount depends on the size of your waffle iron).
7. Cook according to the manufacturer's instructions, usually for about 5 minutes, until golden brown and crisp.
8. Serve warm with your favorite toppings such as fresh fruit, maple syrup, or yogurt.

Tips:

- Make a large batch and freeze extra waffles. Reheat in a toaster for a quick breakfast.
- For a gluten-free version, ensure your oat flour is certified gluten-free.

Pear and Amaranth Pudding

Portions: 2

Ingredients:

- 1/2 cup amaranth
- 1 cup water
- 1 cup pear, diced
- 1 cup coconut milk
- 2 tablespoons maple syrup
- 1 teaspoon vanilla extract
- 1/2 teaspoon cinnamon
- A pinch of salt

Preparation Time: 30 minutes

Nutritional Information (per serving):

Calories	Carbohydrates	Protein	Fat	Fiber	Sugar
250 kcal	40 g	5 g	10 g	5 g	20 g

Instructions:

1. Rinse the amaranth under cold water.
2. In a saucepan, bring the water to a boil. Add the amaranth and reduce to a simmer. Cook for about 20 minutes or until the water is absorbed.
3. Add the diced pear, coconut milk, maple syrup, vanilla extract, cinnamon, and salt to the saucepan.
4. Cook over medium heat, stirring occasionally, for another 10 minutes or until the pudding thickens.
5. Serve warm or chilled, garnished with extra pear slices and a sprinkle of cinnamon.

Tips:

- For a creamier texture, use full-fat coconut milk.
- Add a handful of chopped nuts for extra crunch.

Kamut Toast with Spinach Pesto

Portions: 2

Ingredients:

- 4 slices of Kamut bread
- 2 cups fresh spinach
- 1/4 cup walnuts
- 1/4 cup grated Parmesan cheese
- 1 garlic clove
- 1/4 cup olive oil
- Salt and pepper to taste
- 1 avocado, sliced

Preparation Time: 15 minutes

Nutritional Information (per serving):

Calories	Carbohydrates	Protein	Fat	Fiber	Sugar
350 kcal	40 g	8 g	20 g	7 g	2 g

Instructions:

1. In a food processor, combine spinach, walnuts, Parmesan cheese, and garlic. Pulse until finely chopped.
2. With the food processor running, slowly add the olive oil until the mixture is smooth. Season with salt and pepper to taste.
3. Toast the Kamut bread slices to your desired level of crispiness.
4. Spread the spinach pesto on the toast.
5. Top with avocado slices and serve immediately.

Tips:

- You can store leftover pesto in an airtight container in the fridge for up to a week.
- For added protein, top with a poached egg.

Coconut Yogurt with Nuts and Berries

Portions: 2

Ingredients:

- 2 cups coconut yogurt
- 1/2 cup mixed berries (strawberries, blueberries, raspberries)
- 1/4 cup mixed nuts (almonds, walnuts, cashews)
- 1 tablespoon honey (optional)

Preparation Time: 5 minutes

Nutritional Information (per serving):

Calories	Carbohydrates	Protein	Fat	Fiber	Sugar
220 kcal	20 g	4 g	12 g	6 g	12 g

Instructions:

1. Divide the coconut yogurt between two bowls.
2. Top each bowl with mixed berries and nuts.
3. Drizzle with honey if desired.
4. Serve immediately.

Tips:

- Use granola instead of nuts for added crunch.
- For a dairy-free option, ensure the yogurt is made from coconut milk.

Spiced Teff Porridge

Portions: 2

Ingredients:

- 1/2 cup teff grain
- 1 1/2 cups water
- 1 cup coconut milk
- 1 teaspoon cinnamon
- 1/2 teaspoon ground ginger
- 2 tablespoons maple syrup
- A pinch of salt

Preparation Time: 25 minutes

Nutritional Information (per serving):

Calories	Carbohydrates	Protein	Fat	Fiber	Sugar
290 kcal	45 g	6 g	9 g	6 g	14 g

Instructions:

1. Rinse the teff under cold water.
2. In a saucepan, bring the water to a boil. Add the teff, reduce to a simmer, and cook for about 15 minutes, stirring occasionally.
3. Add the coconut milk, cinnamon, ground ginger, maple syrup, and salt to the saucepan.
4. Cook for another 10 minutes, stirring frequently, until the porridge is thick and creamy.
5. Serve warm, garnished with extra cinnamon or a drizzle of maple syrup.

Tips:

- For added texture, top with chopped nuts or fresh fruit.
- Store leftovers in the fridge and reheat with a splash of milk.

Blueberry Spelt Muffins

Portions: 4

Ingredients:

- 1 1/2 cups spelt flour
- 1/2 cup sugar
- 2 teaspoons baking powder
- 1/2 teaspoon salt
- 1/2 cup almond milk
- 1/4 cup coconut oil, melted
- 2 large eggs
- 1 teaspoon vanilla extract
- 1 cup fresh or frozen blueberries

Preparation Time: 30 minutes

Nutritional Information (per serving):

Calories	Carbohydrates	Protein	Fat	Fiber	Sugar
220 kcal	32 g	5 g	9 g	4 g	12 g

Instructions:

1. Preheat the oven to 350°F (175°C). Line a muffin tin with paper liners.
2. In a large bowl, whisk together the spelt flour, sugar, baking powder, and salt.
3. In another bowl, mix the almond milk, melted coconut oil, eggs, and vanilla extract.
4. Pour the wet ingredients into the dry ingredients and stir until just combined. Gently fold in the blueberries.
5. Divide the batter evenly among the muffin cups.
6. Bake for 20-25 minutes, or until a toothpick inserted into the center comes out clean.
7. Allow to cool in the tin for 10 minutes, then transfer to a wire rack to cool completely.

Tips:

- Use whole spelt flour for a nuttier flavor.
- Add a streusel topping for extra crunch.

Buckwheat and Apricot Pancakes

Portions: 4

Ingredients:

- 1 cup buckwheat flour
- 1/2 cup all-purpose flour
- 2 tablespoons sugar
- 1 tablespoon baking powder
- 1/2 teaspoon salt
- 1 1/4 cups almond milk
- 2 large eggs
- 1/4 cup melted coconut oil
- 1 teaspoon vanilla extract
- 1 cup diced dried apricots

Preparation Time: 20 minutes

Nutritional Information (per serving):

Calories	Carbohydrates	Protein	Fat	Fiber	Sugar
250 kcal	40 g	6 g	8 g	4 g	10 g

Instructions:

1. In a large bowl, whisk together the buckwheat flour, all-purpose flour, sugar, baking powder, and salt.
2. In another bowl, combine the almond milk, eggs, melted coconut oil, and vanilla extract.
3. Pour the wet ingredients into the dry ingredients and stir until just combined. Fold in the diced apricots.
4. Heat a non-stick skillet over medium heat and lightly grease with oil or cooking spray.
5. Pour 1/4 cup of batter onto the skillet for each pancake. Cook until bubbles form on the surface, then flip and cook until golden brown.
6. Serve warm with your favorite toppings, such as maple syrup or fresh fruit.

Tips:

- For extra flavor, soak the dried apricots in orange juice before adding to the batter.
- Keep cooked pancakes warm in a low oven while you finish cooking the rest.

Oatmeal Cream with Fresh Fruit and Nuts

Portions: 2

Ingredients:

- 1 cup rolled oats
- 2 cups water or milk
- 1 tablespoon honey
- 1 teaspoon vanilla extract
- 1/2 teaspoon cinnamon
- 1/4 cup chopped nuts (almonds, walnuts)
- 1/2 cup fresh fruit (berries, banana slices)

Preparation Time: 15 minutes

Nutritional Information (per serving):

Calories	Carbohydrates	Protein	Fat	Fiber	Sugar
300 kcal	45 g	8 g	10 g	7 g	12 g

Instructions:

1. In a saucepan, bring the water or milk to a boil. Stir in the rolled oats, reduce the heat, and simmer for about 5 minutes, stirring occasionally.
2. Remove from heat and stir in honey, vanilla extract, and cinnamon.
3. Divide the oatmeal between two bowls. Top with chopped nuts and fresh fruit.
4. Serve immediately.

Tips:

- Use steel-cut oats for a chewier texture and longer cooking time.
- Add a spoonful of yogurt for extra creaminess.

Blueberry and Spinach Smoothie

Portions: 2

Ingredients:
- 1 cup fresh or frozen blueberries
- 1 cup spinach leaves
- 1 banana
- 1 cup almond milk
- 1 tablespoon chia seeds
- 1 teaspoon honey (optional)
- Ice cubes

Preparation Time: 10 minutes

Nutritional Information (per serving):

Calories	Carbohydrates	Protein	Fat	Fiber	Sugar
180 kcal	30 g	3 g	4 g	6 g	15 g

Instructions:
1. In a blender, combine the blueberries, spinach, banana, almond milk, chia seeds, and honey (if using).
2. Blend until smooth. Add ice cubes and blend again until the ice is crushed.
3. Pour into glasses and serve immediately.

Tips:
- For a protein boost, add a scoop of protein powder.
- Use coconut water instead of almond milk for a lighter smoothie.

Spelt Pancakes

Portions: 4

Ingredients:

- 1 1/2 cups spelt flour
- 2 tablespoons sugar
- 1 tablespoon baking powder
- 1/2 teaspoon salt
- 1 1/2 cups milk (dairy or non-dairy)
- 2 large eggs
- 1/4 cup melted coconut oil
- 1 teaspoon vanilla extract

Preparation Time: 20 minutes

Nutritional Information (per serving):

Calories	Carbohydrates	Protein	Fat	Fiber	Sugar
220 kcal	35 g	6 g	8 g	4 g	8 g

Instructions:

1. In a large bowl, whisk together the spelt flour, sugar, baking powder, and salt.
2. In another bowl, mix the milk, eggs, melted coconut oil, and vanilla extract.
3. Pour the wet ingredients into the dry ingredients and stir until just combined.
4. Heat a non-stick skillet over medium heat and lightly grease with oil or cooking spray.
5. Pour 1/4 cup of batter onto the skillet for each pancake. Cook until bubbles form on the surface, then flip and cook until golden brown.
6. Serve warm with your favorite toppings, such as maple syrup, fresh fruit, or yogurt.

Tips:

- For a fluffier texture, let the batter rest for 10 minutes before cooking.
- Add blueberries or chocolate chips to the batter for extra flavor.

Cinnamon Quinoa Porridge

Portions: 2

Ingredients:

- 1/2 cup quinoa
- 1 cup water
- 1 cup almond milk
- 1 tablespoon honey
- 1 teaspoon vanilla extract
- 1 teaspoon cinnamon
- A pinch of salt

Preparation Time: 25 minutes

Nutritional Information (per serving):

Calories	Carbohydrates	Protein	Fat	Fiber	Sugar
240 kcal	40 g	7 g	6 g	5 g	15 g

Instructions:

1. Rinse the quinoa under cold water.
2. In a saucepan, bring the water to a boil. Add the quinoa, reduce to a simmer, and cook for about 15 minutes until the water is absorbed.
3. Add the almond milk, honey, vanilla extract, cinnamon, and salt to the saucepan.
4. Cook for another 10 minutes, stirring frequently, until the porridge thickens.
5. Serve warm, garnished with a sprinkle of cinnamon or fresh fruit.

Tips:

- For added texture, top with chopped nuts or a dollop of yogurt.
- Store leftovers in the fridge and reheat with a splash of milk.

Kamut Avocado Toast

Portions: 2

Ingredients:

- 4 slices of Kamut bread
- 2 ripe avocados
- 1 tablespoon lemon juice
- Salt and pepper to taste
- Red pepper flakes (optional)
- 1/4 cup cherry tomatoes, halved

Preparation Time: 10 minutes

Nutritional Information (per serving):

Calories	Carbohydrates	Protein	Fat	Fiber	Sugar
300 kcal	35 g	6 g	16 g	8 g	3 g

Instructions:

1. Toast the Kamut bread slices to your desired level of crispiness.
2. In a bowl, mash the avocados with lemon juice, salt, and pepper.
3. Spread the mashed avocado evenly on the toasted bread slices.
4. Top with cherry tomato halves and sprinkle with red pepper flakes if desired.
5. Serve immediately.

Tips:

- Add a poached egg on top for extra protein.
- Drizzle with balsamic glaze for added flavor.

Spelt Banana Muffins

Portions: 4

Ingredients:

- 1 1/2 cups spelt flour
- 1/2 cup sugar
- 1 teaspoon baking soda
- 1/2 teaspoon salt
- 3 ripe bananas, mashed
- 1/3 cup melted coconut oil
- 1 large egg
- 1 teaspoon vanilla extract

Preparation Time: 30 minutes

Nutritional Information (per serving):

Calories	Carbohydrates	Protein	Fat	Fiber	Sugar
230 kcal	35 g	4 g	8 g	4 g	14 g

Instructions:

1. Preheat the oven to 350°F (175°C). Line a muffin tin with paper liners.
2. In a large bowl, whisk together the spelt flour, sugar, baking soda, and salt.
3. In another bowl, mix the mashed bananas, melted coconut oil, egg, and vanilla extract.
4. Pour the wet ingredients into the dry ingredients and stir until just combined.
5. Divide the batter evenly among the muffin cups.
6. Bake for 20-25 minutes, or until a toothpick inserted into the center comes out clean.
7. Allow to cool in the tin for 10 minutes, then transfer to a wire rack to cool completely.

Tips:

- Add chocolate chips or chopped nuts to the batter for extra flavor.
- Store muffins in an airtight container for up to 3 days.

Chia Berry Pudding

Portions: 2

Ingredients:

- 1/4 cup chia seeds
- 1 cup almond milk
- 1 tablespoon honey
- 1/2 teaspoon vanilla extract
- 1/2 cup mixed berries (strawberries, blueberries, raspberries)

Preparation Time: 10 minutes (plus overnight chilling)

Nutritional Information (per serving):

Calories	Carbohydrates	Protein	Fat	Fiber	Sugar
180 kcal	20 g	5 g	9 g	10 g	12 g

Instructions:

1. In a bowl, combine the chia seeds, almond milk, honey, and vanilla extract. Stir well.
2. Cover and refrigerate overnight or for at least 4 hours until the mixture thickens.
3. Stir the pudding before serving and divide between two bowls.
4. Top with mixed berries and serve immediately.

Tips:

- Use coconut milk for a creamier pudding.
- Add a sprinkle of granola for extra crunch.

Tropical Smoothie

Portions: 2

Ingredients:

- 1 cup pineapple chunks
- 1 banana
- 1/2 cup mango chunks
- 1 cup coconut water
- 1 tablespoon chia seeds
- Ice cubes

Preparation Time: 10 minutes

Nutritional Information (per serving):

Calories	Carbohydrates	Protein	Fat	Fiber	Sugar
170 kcal	40 g	2 g	1 g	6 g	28 g

Instructions:

1. In a blender, combine the pineapple chunks, banana, mango chunks, coconut water, and chia seeds.
2. Blend until smooth. Add ice cubes and blend again until the ice is crushed.
3. Pour into glasses and serve immediately.

Tips:

- Use frozen fruit for a thicker, colder smoothie.
- Add a handful of spinach for extra nutrients without changing the flavor.

Alkaline Açaí Bowl

Portions: 2

Ingredients:

- 2 açaí puree packs
- 1 banana
- 1/2 cup almond milk
- 1 tablespoon almond butter
- 1/4 cup granola
- 1/4 cup sliced strawberries
- 1/4 cup blueberries
- 1 tablespoon chia seeds

Preparation Time: 10 minutes

Nutritional Information (per serving):

Calories	Carbohydrates	Protein	Fat	Fiber	Sugar
250 kcal	35 g	6 g	10 g	7 g	20 g

Instructions:

1. In a blender, combine the açaí puree packs, banana, almond milk, and almond butter.
2. Blend until smooth and thick.
3. Divide the mixture between two bowls.
4. Top with granola, sliced strawberries, blueberries, and chia seeds.
5. Serve immediately.

Tips:

- Use frozen banana slices for a thicker consistency.
- Add a drizzle of honey for extra sweetness.

Seed and Nut Energy Bars

Portions: 4

Ingredients:

- 1 cup mixed nuts (almonds, walnuts, cashews)
- 1/2 cup mixed seeds (pumpkin seeds, sunflower seeds, chia seeds)
- 1 cup dates, pitted
- 1/4 cup honey
- 1/4 cup almond butter
- 1 teaspoon vanilla extract
- A pinch of salt

Preparation Time: 20 minutes (plus chilling time)

Nutritional Information (per serving):

Calories	Carbohydrates	Protein	Fat	Fiber	Sugar
300 kcal	35 g	8 g	16 g	7 g	18 g

Instructions:

1. In a food processor, pulse the mixed nuts and seeds until coarsely chopped.
2. Add the dates, honey, almond butter, vanilla extract, and salt. Pulse until the mixture is well combined and sticky.
3. Press the mixture into a lined 8x8-inch baking pan.
4. Chill in the refrigerator for at least 1 hour.
5. Cut into bars and serve.

Tips:

- Store bars in an airtight container in the fridge for up to a week.
- Add chocolate chips for a sweet treat.

Chickpea Flour Vegan Omelette

Portions: 2

Ingredients:

- 1 cup chickpea flour
- 1 cup water
- 1/2 teaspoon turmeric
- 1/2 teaspoon garlic powder
- 1/2 teaspoon salt
- 1/4 teaspoon black pepper
- 1/2 cup diced vegetables (bell peppers, onions, spinach)
- 1 tablespoon olive oil

Preparation Time: 15 minutes

Nutritional Information (per serving):

Calories	Carbohydrates	Protein	Fat	Fiber	Sugar
180 kcal	25 g	8 g	6 g	6 g	3 g

Instructions:

1. In a bowl, whisk together the chickpea flour, water, turmeric, garlic powder, salt, and black pepper until smooth.
2. Heat the olive oil in a non-stick skillet over medium heat.
3. Pour half of the batter into the skillet, spreading it out evenly.
4. Cook for about 2-3 minutes until bubbles form and the edges start to lift.
5. Add half of the diced vegetables on top of the batter.
6. Carefully flip the omelette and cook for another 2-3 minutes until cooked through.
7. Repeat with the remaining batter and vegetables.
8. Serve warm.

Tips:

- Add nutritional yeast for a cheesy flavor.
- Serve with a side of avocado or salsa for extra flavor.

Main Dishes

Farro Salad with Roasted Tomatoes

Portions: 4

Ingredients:

- 1 cup farro
- 2 cups water
- 1 pint cherry tomatoes, halved
- 2 tablespoons olive oil
- Salt and pepper to taste
- 1/4 cup fresh basil, chopped
- 1/4 cup feta cheese, crumbled (optional)
- 2 tablespoons balsamic vinegar

Preparation Time: 30 minutes

Nutritional Information (per serving):

Calories	Carbohydrates	Protein	Fat	Fiber	Sugar
250 kcal	40 g	8 g	8 g	6 g	5 g

Instructions:

1. Preheat the oven to 400°F (200°C).
2. Cook the farro in water according to package instructions. Drain and set aside to cool.
3. Place the cherry tomatoes on a baking sheet, drizzle with 1 tablespoon of olive oil, and season with salt and pepper. Roast for 15 minutes until tender.
4. In a large bowl, combine the cooked farro, roasted tomatoes, basil, and feta cheese (if using).
5. Drizzle with the remaining olive oil and balsamic vinegar. Toss to combine.
6. Serve chilled or at room temperature.

Tips:

- Add chopped cucumbers or olives for extra flavor.
- Use quinoa or barley as an alternative to farro.

Beet and Ginger Soup

Portions: 4

Ingredients:

- 4 medium beets, peeled and diced
- 1 onion, chopped
- 2 tablespoons olive oil
- 1 tablespoon fresh ginger, grated
- 4 cups vegetable broth
- Salt and pepper to taste
- 1/4 cup Greek yogurt (optional)

Preparation Time: 40 minutes

Nutritional Information (per serving):

Calories	Carbohydrates	Protein	Fat	Fiber	Sugar
160 kcal	22 g	4 g	7 g	4 g	10 g

Instructions:

1. In a large pot, heat the olive oil over medium heat. Add the onion and cook until soft, about 5 minutes.
2. Add the beets and ginger, and cook for another 5 minutes.
3. Pour in the vegetable broth and bring to a boil. Reduce heat and simmer for 25 minutes, or until the beets are tender.
4. Use an immersion blender to puree the soup until smooth. Season with salt and pepper.
5. Serve hot, with a dollop of Greek yogurt if desired.

Tips:

- Garnish with fresh herbs like parsley or dill.
- Add a splash of orange juice for a citrusy twist.

Chickpea Flour Crepes with Vegetables

Portions: 4

Ingredients:

- 1 cup chickpea flour
- 1 cup water
- 1/2 teaspoon salt
- 1/4 teaspoon turmeric
- 1/4 teaspoon cumin
- 2 tablespoons olive oil, divided
- 1 cup mixed vegetables (bell peppers, spinach, mushrooms), diced

Preparation Time: 20 minutes

Nutritional Information (per serving):

Calories	Carbohydrates	Protein	Fat	Fiber	Sugar
180 kcal	20 g	6 g	8 g	4 g	3 g

Instructions:

1. In a bowl, whisk together the chickpea flour, water, salt, turmeric, and cumin until smooth.
2. Heat 1 tablespoon of olive oil in a non-stick skillet over medium heat.
3. Pour 1/4 cup of the batter into the skillet, tilting to spread it evenly. Cook for 2-3 minutes until bubbles form and the edges lift.
4. Flip the crepe and cook for another 1-2 minutes. Remove from the skillet and repeat with the remaining batter.
5. In the same skillet, heat the remaining olive oil and sauté the mixed vegetables until tender.
6. Fill each crepe with the sautéed vegetables and serve immediately.

Tips:

- Add a sprinkle of nutritional yeast for a cheesy flavor.
- Serve with a side salad for a complete meal.

Zucchini Spaghetti with Avocado Sauce

Portions: 2

Ingredients:

- 2 large zucchinis, spiralized
- 1 ripe avocado
- 1/4 cup fresh basil leaves
- 1 clove garlic
- 2 tablespoons lemon juice
- 1/4 cup olive oil
- Salt and pepper to taste
- Cherry tomatoes, halved (for garnish)

Preparation Time: 15 minutes

Nutritional Information (per serving):

Calories	Carbohydrates	Protein	Fat	Fiber	Sugar
200 kcal	15 g	3 g	16 g	7 g	5 g

Instructions:

1. In a food processor, combine the avocado, basil, garlic, lemon juice, olive oil, salt, and pepper. Blend until smooth.
2. Toss the zucchini noodles with the avocado sauce until well coated.
3. Garnish with cherry tomatoes and serve immediately.

Tips:

- Add grilled chicken or tofu for extra protein.
- Use a julienne peeler if you don't have a spiralizer.

Quinoa with Asparagus and Toasted Almonds

Portions: 4

Ingredients:

- 1 cup quinoa
- 2 cups water
- 1 bunch asparagus, trimmed and cut into 1-inch pieces
- 1/4 cup sliced almonds, toasted
- 2 tablespoons olive oil
- 1 tablespoon lemon juice
- Salt and pepper to taste

Preparation Time: 25 minutes

Nutritional Information (per serving):

Calories	Carbohydrates	Protein	Fat	Fiber	Sugar
220 kcal	30 g	7 g	9 g	5 g	3 g

Instructions:

1. Rinse the quinoa under cold water.
2. In a saucepan, bring the water to a boil. Add the quinoa, reduce heat, cover, and simmer for 15 minutes until water is absorbed.
3. In another pan, steam the asparagus for 5 minutes until tender-crisp.
4. In a large bowl, combine the cooked quinoa, asparagus, and toasted almonds.
5. Drizzle with olive oil and lemon juice. Season with salt and pepper, and toss to combine.
6. Serve warm or at room temperature.

Tips:

- Add crumbled feta cheese for extra flavor.
- Use other vegetables like peas or broccoli as variations.

Rice Pasta with Cilantro Pesto

Portions: 4

Ingredients:

- 8 oz rice pasta
- 1 bunch fresh cilantro, chopped
- 1/4 cup pine nuts
- 1/4 cup olive oil
- 1 clove garlic
- 2 tablespoons lemon juice
- Salt and pepper to taste
- 1/4 cup grated Parmesan cheese (optional)

Preparation Time: 20 minutes

Nutritional Information (per serving):

Calories	Carbohydrates	Protein	Fat	Fiber	Sugar
280 kcal	40 g	6 g	12 g	3 g	2 g

Instructions:

1. Cook the rice pasta according to package instructions. Drain and set aside.
2. In a food processor, combine the cilantro, pine nuts, olive oil, garlic, lemon juice, salt, and pepper. Blend until smooth.
3. Toss the cooked pasta with the cilantro pesto until well coated.
4. Sprinkle with grated Parmesan cheese if desired, and serve immediately.

Tips:

- Add grilled chicken or shrimp for extra protein.
- Use walnuts or almonds instead of pine nuts.

Millet Risotto with Artichokes

Portions: 4

Ingredients:

- 1 cup millet
- 4 cups vegetable broth
- 1 can artichoke hearts, drained and chopped
- 1 onion, chopped
- 2 tablespoons olive oil
- 1/4 cup white wine (optional)
- 1/4 cup grated Parmesan cheese (optional)
- Salt and pepper to taste

Preparation Time: 30 minutes

Nutritional Information (per serving):

Calories	Carbohydrates	Protein	Fat	Fiber	Sugar
260 kcal	35 g	7 g	10 g	6 g	3 g

Instructions:

1. In a large saucepan, heat the olive oil over medium heat. Add the onion and cook until soft, about 5 minutes.
2. Add the millet and cook for another 2 minutes, stirring frequently.
3. Pour in the white wine (if using) and cook until evaporated.
4. Gradually add the vegetable broth, 1/2 cup at a time, stirring constantly and allowing the liquid to be absorbed before adding more.
5. Stir in the chopped artichokes and cook until the millet is tender, about 20 minutes.
6. Season with salt and pepper. Stir in the Parmesan cheese if desired.
7. Serve warm.

Tips:

- Use fresh artichokes for a more intense flavor.
- Add a squeeze of lemon juice for a bright finish.

Cucumber and Avocado Soup

Portions: 2

Ingredients:

- 2 cucumbers, peeled and chopped
- 1 ripe avocado
- 1/2 cup Greek yogurt
- 1/4 cup fresh dill, chopped
- 1 tablespoon lemon juice
- Salt and pepper to taste
- 1/2 cup water

Preparation Time: 10 minutes

Nutritional Information (per serving):

Calories	Carbohydrates	Protein	Fat	Fiber	Sugar
160 kcal	12 g	5 g	11 g	6 g	5 g

Instructions:

1. In a blender, combine the cucumbers, avocado, Greek yogurt, dill, lemon juice, salt, pepper, and water.
2. Blend until smooth.
3. Chill in the refrigerator for at least 30 minutes before serving.
4. Serve cold, garnished with extra dill if desired.

Tips:

- Add a clove of garlic for a punch of flavor.
- Serve with crusty bread for a complete meal.

Kamut Tagliatelle with Lemon and Thyme

Portions: 2

Ingredients:

- 8 oz Kamut tagliatelle
- 2 tablespoons olive oil
- 1 clove garlic, minced
- 1 tablespoon fresh thyme leaves
- 1 tablespoon lemon zest
- 2 tablespoons lemon juice
- Salt and pepper to taste
- Grated Parmesan cheese (optional)

Preparation Time: 20 minutes

Nutritional Information (per serving):

Calories	Carbohydrates	Protein	Fat	Fiber	Sugar
300 kcal	45 g	8 g	10 g	4 g	2 g

Instructions:

1. Cook the Kamut tagliatelle according to package instructions. Drain and set aside.
2. In a large skillet, heat the olive oil over medium heat. Add the garlic and cook until fragrant, about 1 minute.
3. Add the thyme leaves and lemon zest, cooking for another minute.
4. Toss the cooked tagliatelle in the skillet with the lemon juice, salt, and pepper.
5. Serve warm, garnished with grated Parmesan cheese if desired.

Tips:

- Add a handful of arugula for a peppery flavor.
- Use lime juice and zest for a different citrus twist.

Grilled Vegetable Quinoa Couscous with Tahini

Portions: 4

Ingredients:

- 1 cup quinoa
- 2 cups water
- 1 zucchini, sliced
- 1 bell pepper, sliced
- 1 eggplant, sliced
- 2 tablespoons olive oil
- Salt and pepper to taste
- 2 tablespoons tahini
- 1 tablespoon lemon juice
- 1/4 cup water

Preparation Time: 30 minutes

Nutritional Information (per serving):

Calories	Carbohydrates	Protein	Fat	Fiber	Sugar
270 kcal	35 g	8 g	12 g	6 g	3 g

Instructions:

1. Rinse the quinoa under cold water.
2. In a saucepan, bring the water to a boil. Add the quinoa, reduce heat, cover, and simmer for 15 minutes until water is absorbed.
3. Meanwhile, heat a grill pan over medium-high heat. Toss the zucchini, bell pepper, and eggplant slices with olive oil, salt, and pepper.
4. Grill the vegetables until tender and slightly charred, about 5-7 minutes per side.
5. In a small bowl, whisk together the tahini, lemon juice, and water until smooth.
6. In a large bowl, combine the cooked quinoa and grilled vegetables. Drizzle with the tahini sauce and toss to combine.
7. Serve warm or at room temperature.

Tips:

- Add fresh herbs like parsley or cilantro for extra flavor.
- Use other vegetables like mushrooms or onions as variations.

Quinoa-Stuffed Bell Peppers with Sautéed Mushrooms and Zucchini

Portion Size: Serves 4

Nutritional Information (per serving): Calories: 220, Protein: 8g, Carbohydrates: 36g, Fat: 7g, Fiber: 6g

Ingredients:

- 4 large bell peppers (red, yellow, or orange)
- 1 cup quinoa, rinsed
- 2 cups spring water
- 1 cup mushrooms, chopped
- 1 zucchini, diced
- 1 small onion, diced
- 2 cloves garlic, minced
- 1 tablespoon cold-pressed olive oil
- Fresh herbs (thyme, oregano, or basil)
- Sea salt and cayenne pepper to taste
- 1 tablespoon nutritional yeast (optional, for a cheesy flavor)

Instructions:

1. Preheat the oven to 375°F (190°C). Cut the tops off the bell peppers and remove the seeds and membranes.
2. Cook quinoa in spring water according to package instructions.
3. In a skillet, heat olive oil and sauté onions and garlic until fragrant.
4. Add mushrooms and zucchini, cooking until tender.
5. Mix the cooked quinoa with the sautéed vegetables. Season with sea salt, cayenne pepper, and fresh herbs.
6. Stuff the bell peppers with the quinoa mixture, place them in a baking dish, and cover with foil.
7. Bake for 25-30 minutes until the peppers are tender. Sprinkle with nutritional yeast before serving, if desired.

Tips:

- For added protein, you can mix in some cooked chickpeas or lentils with the quinoa.
- If you prefer a bit more heat, add a pinch of crushed red pepper flakes to the vegetable mixture.
- Leftover stuffing can be used as a side dish or mixed with greens for a salad.

Zucchini Noodles with Avocado Pesto and Cherry Tomatoes

Portion Size: Serves 4

Nutritional Information (per serving): Calories: 290, Protein: 6g, Carbohydrates: 14g, Fat: 26g, Fiber: 9g

Ingredients:

- 4 large zucchinis, spiralized into noodles
- 1 ripe avocado
- 1 cup fresh basil leaves
- 2 cloves garlic
- 1/4 cup cold-pressed olive oil
- 1/4 cup walnuts or pine nuts
- 1 tablespoon fresh lemon juice
- Sea salt and black pepper to taste
- 1 cup cherry tomatoes, halved

Instructions:

1. In a blender, combine avocado, basil leaves, garlic, olive oil, nuts, and lemon juice. Blend until smooth and creamy. Season with sea salt and pepper.
2. Toss the zucchini noodles with the avocado pesto until evenly coated.
3. Add the cherry tomatoes and gently mix.
4. Serve immediately, garnished with extra basil leaves or a sprinkle of walnuts.

Tips:

- For a creamier texture, add a tablespoon of nutritional yeast to the pesto.
- You can also use this pesto as a spread for sandwiches or a dip for vegetables.
- If you don't have a spiralizer, you can use a vegetable peeler to create thin zucchini ribbons.

Butternut Squash and Lentil Curry

Portion Size: Serves 4

Nutritional Information (per serving): Calories: 320, Protein: 13g, Carbohydrates: 52g, Fat: 9g, Fiber: 13g

Ingredients:

- 1 medium butternut squash, peeled and cubed
- 1 cup green or red lentils, rinsed
- 1 can (14 oz) coconut milk
- 2 cups spring water
- 1 onion, diced
- 2 cloves garlic, minced
- 1 tablespoon cold-pressed coconut oil
- 1 tablespoon curry powder
- 1 teaspoon turmeric
- 1 teaspoon ground cumin
- Sea salt and cayenne pepper to taste
- Fresh cilantro, chopped (for garnish)

Instructions:

1. In a large pot, heat coconut oil over medium heat. Sauté onions and garlic until softened.
2. Add curry powder, turmeric, and cumin. Stir to coat the onions and garlic with spices.
3. Add butternut squash cubes, lentils, coconut milk, and water. Stir well and bring to a simmer.
4. Cook for 25-30 minutes until the squash is tender and the lentils are fully cooked, stirring occasionally.
5. Season with sea salt and cayenne pepper.
6. Serve hot, garnished with fresh cilantro.

Tips:

- Serve this curry over a bed of quinoa or spelt grain for a complete meal.
- The curry can be stored in the refrigerator for up to three days and actually tastes better the next day as the flavors meld.
- Add a handful of spinach or kale in the last few minutes of cooking for added nutrients.

Spelt Flour Veggie Tacos

Portion Size: Serves 4 (2 tacos per person)

Nutritional Information (per serving of 2 tacos): Calories: 350, Protein: 12g, Carbohydrates: 52g, Fat: 12g, Fiber: 11g

Ingredients:

- 8 spelt flour tortillas
- 1 cup black beans, cooked
- 1 cup cherry tomatoes, chopped
- 1 avocado, sliced
- 1 red bell pepper, sliced
- 1 cup romaine lettuce, shredded
- 1 small red onion, thinly sliced
- Fresh cilantro, chopped
- Juice of 1 lime
- 2 tablespoons cold-pressed olive oil
- Sea salt and black pepper to taste

Instructions:

1. Warm the spelt tortillas in a dry skillet over medium heat.
2. In a bowl, mix black beans with lime juice, olive oil, sea salt, and black pepper.
3. Assemble the tacos by layering black beans, cherry tomatoes, avocado slices, red bell pepper, romaine lettuce, and red onion on each tortilla.
4. Garnish with fresh cilantro and a squeeze of lime juice before serving.

Tips:

- Add some grilled mushrooms or sautéed zucchini for extra flavor and texture.
- Serve with a side of homemade guacamole or a fresh salsa.
- The spelt tortillas can be made ahead of time and stored in an airtight container.

Baked Plantain and Sweet Potato Medley

Portion Size: Serves 4

Nutritional Information (per serving): Calories: 310, Protein: 3g, Carbohydrates: 58g, Fat: 9g, Fiber: 7g

Ingredients:

- 2 ripe plantains, peeled and sliced into thick rounds
- 2 sweet potatoes, peeled and cubed
- 2 tablespoons cold-pressed olive oil
- 1 teaspoon ground cinnamon
- 1/2 teaspoon ground cumin
- Sea salt and black pepper to taste
- Fresh parsley, chopped (for garnish)

Instructions:

1. Preheat the oven to 400°F (200°C).
2. In a large mixing bowl, toss the plantain slices and sweet potato cubes with olive oil, cinnamon, cumin, sea salt, and black pepper.
3. Spread the mixture in a single layer on a baking sheet.
4. Bake for 25-30 minutes, flipping halfway through, until the sweet potatoes are tender and the plantains are golden and caramelized.
5. Serve warm, garnished with fresh parsley.

Tips:

- This dish pairs well with a side of steamed greens like kale or collard greens.
- For a sweeter version, drizzle a little date syrup over the plantains before serving.
- Leftovers can be reheated in the oven or eaten cold as a salad topping.

Chickpea and Kale Stew

Portion Size: Serves 4

Nutritional Information (per serving): Calories: 280, Protein: 12g, Carbohydrates: 38g, Fat: 10g, Fiber: 10g

Ingredients:

- 1 cup chickpeas, cooked
- 1 bunch kale, chopped
- 1 sweet potato, peeled and diced
- 1 onion, diced
- 2 cloves garlic, minced
- 1 can (14 oz) coconut milk
- 2 cups vegetable broth (alkaline-friendly)
- 1 tablespoon cold-pressed coconut oil
- 1 teaspoon turmeric
- 1 teaspoon cumin
- Sea salt and black pepper to taste
- Fresh cilantro for garnish

Instructions:

1. Heat the coconut oil in a large pot over medium heat. Sauté the onion and garlic until softened.
2. Add the turmeric and cumin, stirring until the onions are well-coated with the spices.
3. Add the sweet potato, chickpeas, coconut milk, and vegetable broth. Bring to a simmer.
4. Cook for 20 minutes, or until the sweet potatoes are tender.
5. Add the chopped kale and cook for an additional 5 minutes until wilted.
6. Season with sea salt and black pepper, and garnish with fresh cilantro before serving.

Tips:

- For a thicker stew, mash some of the sweet potatoes before adding the kale.
- Serve with a side of spelt or quinoa for a more filling meal.
- Leftovers can be refrigerated and taste even better the next day as the flavors deepen.

Spaghetti Squash with Alkaline Marinara Sauce

Portion Size: Serves 4

Nutritional Information (per serving): Calories: 200, Protein: 4g, Carbohydrates: 35g, Fat: 7g, Fiber: 8g

Ingredients:

- 1 large spaghetti squash
- 2 cups cherry tomatoes, halved
- 1 onion, finely chopped
- 2 cloves garlic, minced
- 2 tablespoons cold-pressed olive oil
- 1 tablespoon fresh basil, chopped
- 1 teaspoon oregano
- Sea salt and black pepper to taste
- 1 tablespoon nutritional yeast (optional)

Instructions:

1. Preheat the oven to 400°F (200°C). Cut the spaghetti squash in half lengthwise, remove seeds, and brush with olive oil.
2. Place the squash cut side down on a baking sheet and roast for 40 minutes, or until tender.
3. While the squash is roasting, heat olive oil in a skillet over medium heat. Sauté onions and garlic until fragrant.
4. Add cherry tomatoes, basil, oregano, sea salt, and black pepper. Cook until the tomatoes break down and form a sauce, about 15 minutes.
5. When the squash is done, use a fork to scrape out the strands of squash into a bowl.
6. Top the squash with the marinara sauce and sprinkle with nutritional yeast if desired.

Tips:

- For extra protein, add a handful of cooked chickpeas or lentils to the marinara sauce.
- The squash strands can be sautéed briefly in olive oil for extra flavor before topping with sauce.
- This dish pairs well with a simple green salad or steamed veggies.

Portobello Mushroom Steaks with Garlic and Herbs

Portion Size: Serves 4

Nutritional Information (per serving): Calories: 150, Protein: 5g, Carbohydrates: 8g, Fat: 12g, Fiber: 3g

Ingredients:

- 4 large portobello mushroom caps
- 3 tablespoons cold-pressed olive oil
- 3 cloves garlic, minced
- 1 tablespoon fresh rosemary, chopped
- 1 tablespoon fresh thyme, chopped
- 1 tablespoon balsamic vinegar (optional, as it is mildly acidic)
- Sea salt and black pepper to taste
- Fresh parsley for garnish

Instructions:

1. Preheat the oven to 375°F (190°C).
2. In a small bowl, mix olive oil, garlic, rosemary, thyme, balsamic vinegar (if using), sea salt, and black pepper.
3. Brush the mushroom caps with the mixture, ensuring they are well-coated.
4. Place the mushrooms on a baking sheet and bake for 20-25 minutes until tender.
5. Garnish with fresh parsley before serving.

Tips:

- These mushrooms are perfect as a main dish served with a side of quinoa or a salad.
- For a smoky flavor, grill the mushrooms instead of baking them.
- Leftover mushrooms can be sliced and added to sandwiches or salads.

Alkaline Veggie Stir-Fry with Amaranth

Portion Size: Serves 4

Nutritional Information (per serving): Calories: 290, Protein: 10g, Carbohydrates: 42g, Fat: 9g, Fiber: 8g

Ingredients:

- 1 cup amaranth, rinsed
- 2 cups spring water
- 1 cup broccoli florets
- 1 red bell pepper, sliced
- 1 yellow bell pepper, sliced
- 1 carrot, julienned
- 1 zucchini, sliced
- 2 tablespoons cold-pressed sesame oil
- 2 tablespoons tamari (gluten-free, alkaline-friendly)
- 1 tablespoon fresh ginger, grated
- 2 cloves garlic, minced
- 1 tablespoon sesame seeds
- Sea salt and black pepper to taste

Instructions:

1. Cook the amaranth in 2 cups of spring water, bringing it to a boil and then simmering until the water is absorbed, about 20 minutes.
2. In a large skillet, heat sesame oil over medium heat. Add garlic and ginger, sautéing until fragrant.
3. Add broccoli, bell peppers, carrot, and zucchini. Stir-fry for 5-7 minutes until the vegetables are tender but still crisp.
4. Stir in tamari, sesame seeds, sea salt, and black pepper.
5. Serve the stir-fry over a bed of cooked amaranth.

Tips:

- Add a handful of fresh spinach or kale at the end of cooking for an extra nutrient boost.
- If you prefer more heat, add a pinch of cayenne pepper or a few chili flakes.
- Leftovers make a great cold salad for the next day's lunch.

Stuffed Eggplant with Millet and Herbs

Portion Size: Serves 4

Nutritional Information (per serving): Calories: 310; Protein: 7g, Carbohydrates: 50g, Fat: 10g, Fiber: 11g

Ingredients:

- 2 large eggplants, halved lengthwise
- 1 cup millet, rinsed
- 2 cups vegetable broth (alkaline-friendly)
- 1 onion, finely chopped
- 2 cloves garlic, minced
- 1 cup cherry tomatoes, chopped
- 1 tablespoon fresh mint, chopped
- 1 tablespoon fresh parsley, chopped
- 2 tablespoons cold-pressed olive oil
- Sea salt and black pepper to taste
- 1 tablespoon pine nuts, toasted (optional)

Instructions:

1. Preheat the oven to 375°F (190°C).
2. Scoop out the flesh of the eggplants, leaving a 1/2-inch shell. Chop the eggplant flesh and set aside.
3. In a saucepan, bring vegetable broth to a boil, add millet, and simmer until the liquid is absorbed, about 20 minutes.
4. In a skillet, heat olive oil over medium heat. Sauté onions and garlic until softened.
5. Add the chopped eggplant, tomatoes, mint, and parsley. Cook until the eggplant is tender.
6. Mix the cooked millet with the vegetable mixture. Season with sea salt and black pepper.
7. Stuff the eggplant shells with the millet mixture and place in a baking dish.
8. Cover with foil and bake for 25-30 minutes until the eggplants are tender.
9. Garnish with toasted pine nuts, if using, and serve.

Tips:

- Serve with a side of steamed greens or a fresh salad.
- For added flavor, sprinkle the stuffed eggplants with nutritional yeast before baking.
- Leftover stuffing can be served as a side dish or mixed with greens for a hearty salad.

Main Courses

Adzuki Bean and Sweet Potato Stew

Portions: 4

Ingredients:

- 1 cup adzuki beans, soaked overnight
- 2 medium sweet potatoes, peeled and diced
- 1 onion, chopped
- 2 cloves garlic, minced
- 1-inch piece ginger, grated
- 4 cups vegetable broth
- 1 can diced tomatoes
- 1 tablespoon olive oil
- 1 teaspoon cumin
- 1 teaspoon paprika
- Salt and pepper to taste
- Fresh cilantro for garnish

Preparation Time: 45 minutes

Nutritional Information (per serving):

Calories	Carbohydrates	Protein	Fat	Fiber	Sugar	Sodium
220 kcal	40 g	7 g	4 g	10 g	8 g	480 mg

Instructions:

1. Heat olive oil in a large pot over medium heat. Add the onion, garlic, and ginger. Sauté until fragrant, about 5 minutes.
2. Add the soaked adzuki beans, sweet potatoes, cumin, and paprika. Stir to combine.
3. Pour in the vegetable broth and diced tomatoes. Bring to a boil, then reduce heat and simmer for 30 minutes or until the beans and sweet potatoes are tender.
4. Season with salt and pepper to taste.
5. Garnish with fresh cilantro before serving.

Tips:

- Serve with a side of rice or crusty bread.
- Add a splash of coconut milk for extra creaminess.

Quinoa and Spinach Meatballs

Portions: 4

Ingredients:

- 1 cup quinoa, cooked
- 2 cups fresh spinach, chopped
- 1/2 cup breadcrumbs
- 1/4 cup grated Parmesan cheese
- 1 egg, beaten
- 1 clove garlic, minced
- Salt and pepper to taste
- 2 tablespoons olive oil

Preparation Time: 30 minutes

Nutritional Information (per serving):

Calories	Carbohydrates	Protein	Fat	Fiber	Sugar	Sodium
180 kcal	22 g	7 g	8 g	4 g	2 g	320 mg

Instructions:

1. Preheat the oven to 375°F (190°C). Line a baking sheet with parchment paper.
2. In a large bowl, combine cooked quinoa, chopped spinach, breadcrumbs, Parmesan cheese, beaten egg, garlic, salt, and pepper. Mix well.
3. Form the mixture into 1-inch meatballs and place them on the prepared baking sheet.
4. Brush the meatballs with olive oil.
5. Bake for 20 minutes or until golden brown.
6. Serve warm, with your favorite marinara sauce.

Tips:

- These meatballs can be served over pasta or in a sandwich.
- Freeze any leftovers for a quick meal later.

Sesame Tofu and Broccoli

Portions: 4

Ingredients:

- 1 block firm tofu, drained and cubed
- 2 cups broccoli florets
- 2 tablespoons sesame oil
- 1/4 cup soy sauce
- 1 tablespoon rice vinegar
- 1 tablespoon honey
- 1 clove garlic, minced
- 1 teaspoon grated ginger
- 1 tablespoon sesame seeds

Preparation Time: 20 minutes

Nutritional Information (per serving):

Calories	Carbohydrates	Protein	Fat	Fiber	Sugar	Sodium
200 kcal	12 g	12 g	14 g	4 g	4 g	540 mg

Instructions:

1. Heat sesame oil in a large skillet over medium-high heat. Add tofu cubes and cook until golden brown on all sides, about 5-7 minutes.
2. Remove tofu from the skillet and set aside.
3. In the same skillet, add broccoli florets and cook until tender-crisp, about 5 minutes.
4. In a small bowl, whisk together soy sauce, rice vinegar, honey, garlic, and ginger.
5. Return tofu to the skillet and pour the sauce over the tofu and broccoli. Stir to coat.
6. Sprinkle with sesame seeds and serve immediately.

Tips:

- Serve over rice or noodles for a complete meal.
- Add a pinch of red pepper flakes for a bit of heat.

Green Curry Vegetables with Cauliflower Rice

Portions: 4

Ingredients:

- 1 tablespoon coconut oil
- 1 onion, chopped
- 2 cloves garlic, minced
- 1-inch piece ginger, grated
- 2 tablespoons green curry paste
- 1 can coconut milk
- 1 red bell pepper, sliced
- 1 zucchini, sliced
- 1 cup snap peas
- 1 head cauliflower, riced
- Salt and pepper to taste
- Fresh cilantro for garnish

Preparation Time: 30 minutes

Nutritional Information (per serving):

Calories	Carbohydrates	Protein	Fat	Fiber	Sugar	Sodium
250 kcal	20 g	6 g	18 g	6 g	6 g	400 mg

Instructions:

1. In a large skillet, heat coconut oil over medium heat. Add onion, garlic, and ginger. Sauté until fragrant, about 5 minutes.
2. Stir in green curry paste and cook for another minute.
3. Add coconut milk, red bell pepper, zucchini, and snap peas. Simmer for 10 minutes until vegetables are tender.
4. Meanwhile, cook cauliflower rice in a separate pan until tender, about 5 minutes. Season with salt and pepper.
5. Serve the green curry vegetables over the cauliflower rice. Garnish with fresh cilantro.

Tips:

- Adjust the level of curry paste to your taste preference.
- Add tofu or chickpeas for extra protein.

Lentil and Squash Casserole

Portions: 4

Ingredients:

- 1 cup green lentils
- 1 butternut squash, peeled and diced
- 1 onion, chopped
- 2 cloves garlic, minced
- 2 cups vegetable broth
- 1 teaspoon thyme
- 1 teaspoon rosemary
- 2 tablespoons olive oil
- Salt and pepper to taste
- 1/2 cup grated Parmesan cheese (optional)

Preparation Time: 40 minutes

Nutritional Information (per serving):

Calories	Carbohydrates	Protein	Fat	Fiber	Sugar	Sodium
280 kcal	40 g	10 g	8 g	10 g	8 g	420 mg

Instructions:

1. Preheat the oven to 375°F (190°C).
2. In a large skillet, heat olive oil over medium heat. Add onion and garlic, sauté until soft, about 5 minutes.
3. Add diced butternut squash, thyme, and rosemary. Cook for 5 minutes.
4. Stir in green lentils and vegetable broth. Bring to a boil, then reduce heat and simmer for 20 minutes until lentils are tender.
5. Transfer the mixture to a baking dish. Sprinkle with grated Parmesan cheese if using.
6. Bake for 15 minutes until the top is golden brown.
7. Serve warm.

Tips:

- Use sweet potatoes instead of butternut squash for a different flavor.
- Add a handful of spinach before baking for extra greens.

Vegetable Fajitas with Coconut Flour Tortillas

Portions: 4

Ingredients:

- 2 bell peppers, sliced
- 1 onion, sliced
- 1 zucchini, sliced
- 2 tablespoons olive oil
- 1 teaspoon cumin
- 1 teaspoon paprika
- Salt and pepper to taste
- 1/2 cup coconut flour
- 2 tablespoons psyllium husk
- 1/4 teaspoon baking powder
- 1/4 teaspoon salt
- 1 cup warm water

Preparation Time: 25 minutes

Nutritional Information (per serving):

Calories	Carbohydrates	Protein	Fat	Fiber	Sugar	Sodium
200 kcal	20 g	5 g	10 g	10 g	5 g	320 mg

Instructions:

1. In a large skillet, heat olive oil over medium-high heat. Add bell peppers, onion, and zucchini. Cook until tender, about 10 minutes.
2. Season with cumin, paprika, salt, and pepper.
3. In a bowl, mix coconut flour, psyllium husk, baking powder, and salt. Add warm water and stir until a dough forms.
4. Divide the dough into 4 balls. Roll out each ball between two sheets of parchment paper to form tortillas.
5. Cook each tortilla in a dry skillet over medium heat for 2-3 minutes per side.
6. Serve the vegetable fajitas with the coconut flour tortillas.

Tips:

- Add avocado slices or guacamole for extra flavor.
- Use other vegetables like mushrooms or corn as variations.

Portobello Mushroom and Quinoa Burger

Portions: 4

Ingredients:

- 4 large portobello mushrooms
- 1 cup cooked quinoa
- 1/2 cup breadcrumbs
- 1/4 cup grated Parmesan cheese
- 1 egg, beaten
- 1 clove garlic, minced
- 1 tablespoon olive oil
- Salt and pepper to taste
- Burger buns and desired toppings

Preparation Time: 30 minutes

Nutritional Information (per serving):

Calories	Carbohydrates	Protein	Fat	Fiber	Sugar	Sodium
250 kcal	30 g	10 g	10 g	5 g	3 g	400 mg

Instructions:

1. Preheat the oven to 375°F (190°C). Line a baking sheet with parchment paper.
2. In a large bowl, combine cooked quinoa, breadcrumbs, Parmesan cheese, beaten egg, garlic, salt, and pepper.
3. Remove the stems from the portobello mushrooms and fill the caps with the quinoa mixture.
4. Place the mushrooms on the prepared baking sheet and brush with olive oil.
5. Bake for 20 minutes until the mushrooms are tender and the filling is golden brown.
6. Serve on burger buns with your favorite toppings.

Tips:

- Add a slice of cheese or avocado to the burger.
- Serve with sweet potato fries for a complete meal.

Sweet and Sour Tempeh with Pineapple

Portions: 4

Ingredients:

- 1 block tempeh, cubed
- 1 cup pineapple chunks
- 1 bell pepper, sliced
- 1 onion, sliced
- 1/4 cup soy sauce
- 1/4 cup rice vinegar
- 2 tablespoons honey
- 1 tablespoon ketchup
- 2 tablespoons olive oil
- 1 tablespoon cornstarch mixed with 2 tablespoons water
- Salt and pepper to taste

Preparation Time: 25 minutes

Nutritional Information (per serving):

Calories	Carbohydrates	Protein	Fat	Fiber	Sugar	Sodium
280 kcal	30 g	12 g	12 g	4 g	15 g	540 mg

Instructions:

1. In a large skillet, heat olive oil over medium-high heat. Add tempeh cubes and cook until golden brown, about 5-7 minutes.
2. Add bell pepper and onion, cooking until tender, about 5 minutes.
3. Stir in pineapple chunks, soy sauce, rice vinegar, honey, and ketchup. Cook for 2 minutes.
4. Add the cornstarch mixture to the skillet and stir until the sauce thickens.
5. Season with salt and pepper to taste.
6. Serve warm over rice.

Tips:

- Add a pinch of red pepper flakes for a bit of heat.
- Use tofu instead of tempeh if preferred.

Sweet Potato and Kale Gratin

Portions: 4

Ingredients:

- 2 large sweet potatoes, peeled and thinly sliced
- 2 cups kale, chopped
- 1 cup coconut milk
- 1/2 cup vegetable broth
- 1/4 cup nutritional yeast
- 2 cloves garlic, minced
- Salt and pepper to taste
- 1 tablespoon olive oil

Preparation Time: 45 minutes

Nutritional Information (per serving):

Calories	Carbohydrates	Protein	Fat	Fiber	Sugar	Sodium
240 kcal	35 g	5 g	10 g	6 g	8 g	360 mg

Instructions:

1. Preheat the oven to 375°F (190°C). Grease a baking dish with olive oil.
2. In a large bowl, mix sweet potato slices, chopped kale, coconut milk, vegetable broth, nutritional yeast, garlic, salt, and pepper.
3. Layer the sweet potato and kale mixture in the prepared baking dish.
4. Cover with foil and bake for 30 minutes. Remove foil and bake for an additional 15 minutes until the top is golden brown and the sweet potatoes are tender.
5. Serve warm.

Tips:

- Add a sprinkle of grated cheese on top before baking for extra richness.
- Serve as a side dish with grilled protein.

Warm Chickpea and Roasted Vegetable Salad

Portions: 4

Ingredients:

- 1 can chickpeas, drained and rinsed
- 1 red bell pepper, diced
- 1 zucchini, diced
- 1 red onion, diced
- 2 tablespoons olive oil
- 1 teaspoon cumin
- 1 teaspoon paprika
- Salt and pepper to taste
- 1 tablespoon lemon juice
- Fresh parsley for garnish

Preparation Time: 25 minutes

Nutritional Information (per serving):

Calories	Carbohydrates	Protein	Fat	Fiber	Sugar	Sodium
180 kcal	25 g	6 g	7 g	6 g	6 g	320 mg

Instructions:

1. Preheat the oven to 400°F (200°C). Line a baking sheet with parchment paper.
2. In a large bowl, toss chickpeas, bell pepper, zucchini, and red onion with olive oil, cumin, paprika, salt, and pepper.
3. Spread the mixture on the prepared baking sheet and roast for 20 minutes until vegetables are tender and slightly charred.
4. Transfer the roasted vegetables and chickpeas to a large bowl. Drizzle with lemon juice and toss to combine.
5. Garnish with fresh parsley before serving.

Tips:

- Serve over a bed of mixed greens for a heartier salad.
- Add a dollop of hummus for extra flavor.

Quinoa-Stuffed Bell Peppers with Alkaline Pesto

Portion Size: Serves 4

Nutritional Information (per serving): Calories: 350, Protein: 12g, Carbohydrates: 48g, Fat: 13g, Fiber: 9g

Ingredients:

- 4 large bell peppers (any color)
- 1 cup quinoa, rinsed
- 2 cups vegetable broth (alkaline-friendly)
- 1 zucchini, diced
- 1 cup cherry tomatoes, halved
- 1/4 cup red onion, finely chopped
- 1/4 cup pine nuts (or sunflower seeds)
- 2 tablespoons cold-pressed olive oil
- 1/4 cup fresh basil leaves
- 2 cloves garlic, minced
- Sea salt and black pepper to taste
- Fresh parsley for garnish

Instructions:

1. Preheat the oven to 375°F (190°C). Cut the tops off the bell peppers and remove the seeds.
2. Cook the quinoa in vegetable broth according to package instructions, then set aside.
3. In a skillet, heat olive oil over medium heat. Sauté the zucchini, cherry tomatoes, and red onion until tender.
4. Mix the cooked quinoa with the sautéed vegetables and season with sea salt and black pepper.
5. Stuff the bell peppers with the quinoa mixture and place them in a baking dish.
6. Cover with foil and bake for 25-30 minutes until the peppers are tender.
7. Meanwhile, prepare the pesto by blending the basil leaves, garlic, pine nuts, and a pinch of sea salt in a food processor until smooth.
8. Drizzle the stuffed peppers with the pesto and garnish with fresh parsley before serving.

Tips:

- For added flavor, you can roast the bell peppers before stuffing them.
- This dish pairs well with a light salad or a side of steamed greens.
- The quinoa stuffing can be prepared ahead of time and stored in the fridge.

Butternut Squash and Lentil Curry

Portion Size: Serves 4

Nutritional Information (per serving): Calories: 320, Protein: 14g, Carbohydrates: 55g, Fat: 8g, Fiber: 14g

Ingredients:

- 1 butternut squash, peeled and cubed
- 1 cup lentils, rinsed
- 1 can (14 oz) coconut milk
- 2 cups vegetable broth (alkaline-friendly)
- 1 onion, chopped
- 2 cloves garlic, minced
- 1 tablespoon curry powder
- 1 teaspoon turmeric
- 1 tablespoon cold-pressed coconut oil
- Sea salt and black pepper to taste
- Fresh cilantro for garnish

Instructions:

1. In a large pot, heat coconut oil over medium heat. Sauté the onion and garlic until softened.
2. Add curry powder and turmeric, stirring to coat the onions and garlic.
3. Add butternut squash, lentils, coconut milk, and vegetable broth. Bring to a simmer.
4. Cook for 25-30 minutes, or until the lentils and squash are tender.
5. Season with sea salt and black pepper. Garnish with fresh cilantro before serving.

Tips:

- Serve this curry over a bed of quinoa or wild rice for a complete meal.
- For a spicier curry, add a pinch of cayenne pepper or chopped chili.
- Leftovers can be frozen and reheated for a quick meal later on.

Spelt Pasta with Alkaline Alfredo Sauce

Portion Size: Serves 4

Nutritional Information (per serving): Calories: 380, Protein: 15g, Carbohydrates: 60g, Fat: 10g, Fiber: 9g

Ingredients:

- 8 oz spelt pasta
- 1/2 cup raw cashews, soaked for 4 hours
- 1 cup spring water
- 1/4 cup nutritional yeast
- 2 cloves garlic, minced
- 1 tablespoon cold-pressed olive oil
- 1 tablespoon lemon juice
- 1 teaspoon sea salt
- Fresh parsley for garnish

Instructions:

1. Cook the spelt pasta according to package instructions. Drain and set aside.
2. In a blender, combine soaked cashews, spring water, nutritional yeast, garlic, olive oil, lemon juice, and sea salt. Blend until smooth and creamy.
3. Pour the cashew Alfredo sauce over the cooked pasta and toss to combine.
4. Garnish with fresh parsley before serving.

Tips:

- Add steamed broccoli or sautéed mushrooms to the pasta for extra nutrients.
- This sauce can also be used as a creamy base for other dishes, such as casseroles or baked vegetables.
- The Alfredo sauce can be made ahead of time and stored in the fridge for up to 3 days.

Grilled Vegetable Skewers with Spicy Tahini Sauce

Portion Size: Serves 4

Nutritional Information (per serving): Calories: 290, Protein: 8g, Carbohydrates: 35g, Fat: 15g, Fiber: 10g

Ingredients:

- 2 zucchinis, sliced into rounds
- 1 red bell pepper, cut into chunks
- 1 yellow bell pepper, cut into chunks
- 1 red onion, cut into wedges
- 8 oz mushrooms, halved
- 2 tablespoons cold-pressed olive oil
- 1 teaspoon sea salt
- 1 teaspoon black pepper
- 1/4 cup tahini
- 2 tablespoons lemon juice
- 1 tablespoon tamari (gluten-free, alkaline-friendly)
- 1 teaspoon cayenne pepper
- Spring water, as needed for thinning

Instructions:

1. Preheat the grill to medium heat.
2. In a large bowl, toss the vegetables with olive oil, sea salt, and black pepper.
3. Thread the vegetables onto skewers and grill for 10-12 minutes, turning occasionally, until the vegetables are tender and slightly charred.
4. Meanwhile, prepare the spicy tahini sauce by whisking together tahini, lemon juice, tamari, cayenne pepper, and enough spring water to reach the desired consistency.
5. Drizzle the grilled vegetables with the spicy tahini sauce before serving.

Tips:

- Serve these skewers with a side of quinoa or wild rice for a more filling meal.
- The tahini sauce can also be used as a dressing for salads or a dip for raw vegetables.
- For added flavor, marinate the vegetables in the sauce for an hour before grilling.

Zucchini Noodles with Avocado Basil Sauce

Portion Size: Serves 4

Nutritional Information (per serving): Calories: 310, Protein: 6g, Carbohydrates: 20g, Fat: 24g, Fiber: 10g

Ingredients:

- 4 large zucchinis, spiralized into noodles
- 2 ripe avocados
- 1/4 cup fresh basil leaves
- 2 cloves garlic
- 2 tablespoons lemon juice
- 2 tablespoons cold-pressed olive oil
- Sea salt and black pepper to taste
- Cherry tomatoes, halved (optional, for garnish)
- Hemp seeds (optional, for garnish)

Instructions:

1. Spiralize the zucchinis into noodles and set aside.
2. In a blender, combine avocados, basil, garlic, lemon juice, olive oil, sea salt, and black pepper. Blend until smooth and creamy.
3. Toss the zucchini noodles with the avocado basil sauce until well coated.
4. Garnish with cherry tomatoes and hemp seeds if desired, and serve immediately.

Tips:

- This dish is best served fresh as the zucchini noodles may release water if stored for too long.
- Add a handful of baby spinach or arugula for extra greens.
- For a heartier meal, mix in some cooked quinoa or grilled portobello mushrooms.

Sides

Roasted Cauliflower with Paprika

Portions: 4

Ingredients:

- 1 large head of cauliflower, cut into florets
- 2 tablespoons olive oil
- 1 teaspoon paprika
- 1/2 teaspoon garlic powder
- Salt and pepper to taste

Preparation Time: 30 minutes

Nutritional Information (per serving):

Calories	Carbohydrates	Protein	Fat	Fiber	Sugar	Sodium
120 kcal	12 g	4 g	8 g	5 g	3 g	220 mg

Instructions:

1. Preheat the oven to 400°F (200°C). Line a baking sheet with parchment paper.
2. In a large bowl, toss cauliflower florets with olive oil, paprika, garlic powder, salt, and pepper.
3. Spread the cauliflower in a single layer on the prepared baking sheet.
4. Roast for 25-30 minutes, until the cauliflower is tender and golden brown, stirring halfway through.
5. Serve warm.

Tips:

- Add a squeeze of lemon juice before serving for extra flavor.
- Serve as a side dish with your favorite protein.

Rosemary Roasted Potatoes

Portions: 4

Ingredients:

- 4 medium potatoes, diced
- 2 tablespoons olive oil
- 1 tablespoon fresh rosemary, chopped
- Salt and pepper to taste

Preparation Time: 40 minutes

Nutritional Information (per serving):

Calories	Carbohydrates	Protein	Fat	Fiber	Sugar	Sodium
180 kcal	30 g	4 g	6 g	4 g	2 g	300 mg

Instructions:

1. Preheat the oven to 425°F (220°C). Line a baking sheet with parchment paper.
2. In a large bowl, toss diced potatoes with olive oil, rosemary, salt, and pepper.
3. Spread the potatoes in a single layer on the prepared baking sheet.
4. Roast for 35-40 minutes, until the potatoes are golden brown and crispy, stirring halfway through.
5. Serve warm.

Tips:

- Add minced garlic for extra flavor.
- Serve with a dollop of sour cream or Greek yogurt.

Avocado and Tomato Salad

Portions: 4

Ingredients:

- 2 ripe avocados, diced
- 1 cup cherry tomatoes, halved
- 1/4 cup red onion, finely chopped
- 2 tablespoons fresh lime juice
- 1 tablespoon olive oil
- Salt and pepper to taste
- Fresh cilantro for garnish

Preparation Time: 10 minutes

Nutritional Information (per serving):

Calories	Carbohydrates	Protein	Fat	Fiber	Sugar	Sodium
220 kcal	12 g	3 g	20 g	8 g	3 g	150 mg

Instructions:

1. In a large bowl, combine diced avocados, cherry tomatoes, and red onion.
2. Drizzle with lime juice and olive oil.
3. Season with salt and pepper to taste.
4. Toss gently to combine.
5. Garnish with fresh cilantro before serving.

Tips:

- Add diced cucumber for extra crunch.
- Serve as a side dish or as a topping for grilled chicken or fish.

Steamed Broccoli with Almond Sauce

Portions: 4

Ingredients:

- 1 large head of broccoli, cut into florets
- 1/4 cup almond butter
- 2 tablespoons soy sauce
- 1 tablespoon rice vinegar
- 1 tablespoon honey
- 1 clove garlic, minced
- 1 teaspoon grated ginger
- Water, as needed

Preparation Time: 15 minutes

Nutritional Information (per serving):

Calories	Carbohydrates	Protein	Fat	Fiber	Sugar	Sodium
180 kcal	14 g	6 g	12 g	5 g	4 g	400 mg

Instructions:

1. Steam the broccoli florets until tender, about 5-7 minutes.
2. In a small bowl, whisk together almond butter, soy sauce, rice vinegar, honey, garlic, and ginger. Add water as needed to reach a smooth consistency.
3. Drizzle the almond sauce over the steamed broccoli.
4. Serve warm.

Tips:

- Garnish with toasted sesame seeds for extra flavor.
- Serve as a side dish with Asian-inspired meals.

Lemon and Mint Cucumber Salad

Portions: 4

Ingredients:

- 2 large cucumbers, thinly sliced
- 1/4 cup fresh mint leaves, chopped
- 2 tablespoons fresh lemon juice
- 1 tablespoon olive oil
- Salt and pepper to taste

Preparation Time: 10 minutes

Nutritional Information (per serving):

Calories	Carbohydrates	Protein	Fat	Fiber	Sugar	Sodium
60 kcal	6 g	1 g	4 g	2 g	2 g	50 mg

Instructions:

1. In a large bowl, combine sliced cucumbers and chopped mint leaves.
2. Drizzle with lemon juice and olive oil.
3. Season with salt and pepper to taste.
4. Toss gently to combine.
5. Serve chilled.

Tips:

- Add sliced red onions for extra flavor.
- Serve as a refreshing side dish for summer barbecues.

Grilled Zucchini with Basil

Portions: 4

Ingredients:

- 4 medium zucchinis, sliced lengthwise
- 2 tablespoons olive oil
- 1/4 cup fresh basil leaves, chopped
- Salt and pepper to taste

Preparation Time: 15 minutes

Nutritional Information (per serving):

Calories	Carbohydrates	Protein	Fat	Fiber	Sugar	Sodium
90 kcal	6 g	2 g	7 g	2 g	4 g	120 mg

Instructions:

1. Preheat the grill to medium-high heat.
2. Brush zucchini slices with olive oil and season with salt and pepper.
3. Grill the zucchini slices for 2-3 minutes on each side, until tender and charred.
4. Remove from the grill and sprinkle with fresh basil leaves.
5. Serve warm.

Tips:

- Add a squeeze of lemon juice before serving.
- Pair with grilled meats or fish.

Carrot and Walnut Salad

Portions: 4

Ingredients:

- 4 large carrots, grated
- 1/2 cup walnuts, chopped
- 1/4 cup raisins
- 2 tablespoons fresh lemon juice
- 1 tablespoon olive oil
- Salt and pepper to taste

Preparation Time: 10 minutes

Nutritional Information (per serving):

Calories	Carbohydrates	Protein	Fat	Fiber	Sugar	Sodium
180 kcal	20 g	3 g	10 g	4 g	8 g	50 mg

Instructions:

1. In a large bowl, combine grated carrots, chopped walnuts, and raisins.
2. Drizzle with lemon juice and olive oil.
3. Season with salt and pepper to taste.
4. Toss gently to combine.
5. Serve chilled.

Tips:

- Add a pinch of cinnamon for extra flavor.
- Serve as a side dish or light snack.

Sautéed Spinach with Garlic and Lemon

Portions: 4

Ingredients:

- 1 pound fresh spinach
- 2 tablespoons olive oil
- 3 cloves garlic, minced
- 1 tablespoon fresh lemon juice
- Salt and pepper to taste

Preparation Time: 10 minutes

Nutritional Information (per serving):

Calories	Carbohydrates	Protein	Fat	Fiber	Sugar	Sodium
90 kcal	4 g	2 g	7 g	2 g	1 g	120 mg

Instructions:

1. Heat olive oil in a large skillet over medium heat. Add minced garlic and sauté until fragrant, about 1 minute.
2. Add fresh spinach to the skillet and cook until wilted, about 3-5 minutes.
3. Drizzle with lemon juice and season with salt and pepper to taste.
4. Serve warm.

Tips:

- Add a pinch of red pepper flakes for a bit of heat.
- Serve as a side dish with pasta or grilled meats.

Marinated Beetroot

Portions: 4

Ingredients:

- 4 medium beetroots, cooked and sliced
- 1/4 cup apple cider vinegar
- 2 tablespoons olive oil
- 1 tablespoon honey
- 1 teaspoon Dijon mustard
- Salt and pepper to taste
- Fresh dill for garnish

Preparation Time: 15 minutes + marinating time

Nutritional Information (per serving):

Calories	Carbohydrates	Protein	Fat	Fiber	Sugar	Sodium
100 kcal	15 g	2 g	4 g	4 g	11 g	140 mg

Instructions:

1. In a small bowl, whisk together apple cider vinegar, olive oil, honey, Dijon mustard, salt, and pepper.
2. Place cooked and sliced beetroots in a large bowl. Pour the dressing over the beetroots and toss to coat.
3. Cover and refrigerate for at least 1 hour to marinate.
4. Garnish with fresh dill before serving.

Tips:

- Use golden beetroots for a colorful variation.
- Serve as a side dish or salad topping.

Sautéed Asparagus and Mushrooms

Portions: 4

Ingredients:

- 1 bunch asparagus, trimmed and cut into 2-inch pieces
- 1 cup mushrooms, sliced
- 2 tablespoons olive oil
- 2 cloves garlic, minced
- Salt and pepper to taste

Preparation Time: 15 minutes

Nutritional Information (per serving):

Calories	Carbohydrates	Protein	Fat	Fiber	Sugar	Sodium
100 kcal	8 g	3 g	7 g	3 g	2 g	140 mg

Instructions:

1. Heat olive oil in a large skillet over medium heat. Add minced garlic and sauté until fragrant, about 1 minute.
2. Add asparagus and mushrooms to the skillet. Cook until tender, about 5-7 minutes.
3. Season with salt and pepper to taste.
4. Serve warm.

Tips:

- Add a splash of balsamic vinegar for extra flavor.
- Serve as a side dish with grilled proteins.

Desserts

Mango Chia Seed Panna Cotta

Portions: 4

Ingredients:

- 1 ripe mango, peeled and diced
- 1 cup coconut milk
- 2 tablespoons chia seeds
- 2 tablespoons honey (or maple syrup)
- 1 teaspoon vanilla extract

Preparation Time: 15 minutes + chilling time

Nutritional Information (per serving):

Calories	Carbohydrates	Protein	Fat	Fiber	Sugar	Sodium
160 kcal	18 g	2 g	9 g	4 g	12 g	25 mg

Instructions:

1. Blend the diced mango, coconut milk, honey, and vanilla extract until smooth.
2. Stir in the chia seeds.
3. Pour the mixture into serving cups.
4. Refrigerate for at least 4 hours or until set.
5. Serve chilled, garnished with fresh mango slices.

Tips:

- Use frozen mango for a thicker consistency.
- Top with shredded coconut or mint leaves for extra flavor.

Avocado and Chocolate Brownies

Pieces: 8

Ingredients:

- 1 ripe avocado, mashed
- 1 cup almond flour
- 1/2 cup cocoa powder
- 1/2 cup maple syrup
- 1 teaspoon baking soda
- 1 teaspoon vanilla extract
- 2 large eggs (or flax eggs for vegan option)
- 1/2 cup dark chocolate chips

Preparation Time: 35 minutes

Nutritional Information (per serving):

Calories	Carbohydrates	Protein	Fat	Fiber	Sugar	Sodium
200 kcal	18 g	4 g	14 g	4 g	10 g	120 mg

Instructions:

1. Preheat the oven to 350°F (175°C). Line an 8x8-inch baking pan with parchment paper.
2. In a large bowl, mix mashed avocado, almond flour, cocoa powder, maple syrup, baking soda, vanilla extract, and eggs until smooth.
3. Fold in the dark chocolate chips.
4. Pour the batter into the prepared baking pan.
5. Bake for 25-30 minutes, or until a toothpick inserted into the center comes out clean.
6. Allow to cool before cutting into squares.

Tips:

- Store in the fridge for a fudgier texture.
- Add a sprinkle of sea salt on top before baking for a sweet and salty combo.

Lemon and Basil Sorbet

Portions: 4

Ingredients:

- 1 cup fresh lemon juice (about 4-5 lemons)
- 1 cup water
- 1/2 cup honey (or agave syrup)
- 1/4 cup fresh basil leaves, chopped

Preparation Time: 10 minutes + freezing time

Nutritional Information (per serving):

Calories	Carbohydrates	Protein	Fat	Fiber	Sugar	Sodium
100 kcal	27 g	1 g	0 g	1 g	25 g	5 mg

Instructions:

1. In a saucepan, combine water and honey. Heat until the honey is dissolved, then remove from heat.
2. Stir in the fresh lemon juice and chopped basil leaves.
3. Pour the mixture into a shallow dish and freeze until solid, about 4-6 hours.
4. Scrape with a fork to form a slush and serve immediately.

Tips:

- Garnish with lemon zest or extra basil leaves.
- Use an ice cream maker for a smoother texture.

Alkaline Apple Cake

Portions: 8

Ingredients:

- 2 cups spelt flour
- 1 cup unsweetened applesauce
- 1/2 cup coconut sugar
- 1/4 cup coconut oil, melted
- 1 teaspoon baking soda
- 1 teaspoon cinnamon
- 1/2 teaspoon nutmeg
- 1/2 teaspoon salt
- 1 teaspoon vanilla extract
- 1/4 cup chopped walnuts (optional)

Preparation Time: 45 minutes

Nutritional Information (per serving):

Calories	Carbohydrates	Protein	Fat	Fiber	Sugar	Sodium
180 kcal	30 g	3 g	7 g	4 g	15 g	200 mg

Instructions:

1. Preheat the oven to 350°F (175°C). Grease a 9-inch round cake pan.
2. In a large bowl, mix together spelt flour, coconut sugar, baking soda, cinnamon, nutmeg, and salt.
3. Add applesauce, melted coconut oil, and vanilla extract. Stir until well combined.
4. Fold in chopped walnuts, if using.
5. Pour the batter into the prepared cake pan.
6. Bake for 30-35 minutes, or until a toothpick inserted into the center comes out clean.
7. Allow to cool before serving.

Tips:

- Top with a dusting of powdered sugar or a dollop of coconut whipped cream.
- Serve with fresh apple slices for extra flavor.

Lemon Poppy Seed Muffins

Pieces: 12

Ingredients:

- 2 cups spelt flour
- 1/2 cup coconut sugar
- 1/4 cup poppy seeds
- 1 teaspoon baking powder
- 1/2 teaspoon baking soda
- 1/4 teaspoon salt
- 1 cup almond milk
- 1/4 cup coconut oil, melted
- 2 large eggs (or flax eggs for vegan option)
- 1/4 cup fresh lemon juice
- 1 tablespoon lemon zest

Preparation Time: 25 minutes

Nutritional Information (per serving):

Calories	Carbohydrates	Protein	Fat	Fiber	Sugar	Sodium
150 kcal	20 g	4 g	7 g	2 g	10 g	160 mg

Instructions:

1. Preheat the oven to 375°F (190°C). Line a muffin tin with paper liners.
2. In a large bowl, mix spelt flour, coconut sugar, poppy seeds, baking powder, baking soda, and salt.
3. In another bowl, whisk almond milk, melted coconut oil, eggs, lemon juice, and lemon zest.
4. Pour the wet ingredients into the dry ingredients and stir until just combined.
5. Divide the batter evenly among the muffin cups.
6. Bake for 20-25 minutes, or until a toothpick inserted into the center comes out clean.
7. Allow to cool before serving.

Tips:

- Add a lemon glaze made from powdered sugar and lemon juice.
- Store in an airtight container for up to 3 days.

Almond and Ginger Cookies

Pieces: 24

Ingredients:

- 2 cups almond flour
- 1/2 cup coconut sugar
- 1/4 cup coconut oil, melted
- 1 large egg (or flax egg for vegan option)
- 1 tablespoon fresh ginger, grated
- 1 teaspoon vanilla extract
- 1/2 teaspoon baking soda
- 1/4 teaspoon salt

Preparation Time: 20 minutes

Nutritional Information (per serving):

Calories	Carbohydrates	Protein	Fat	Fiber	Sugar	Sodium
90 kcal	6 g	2 g	7 g	1 g	4 g	50 mg

Instructions:

1. Preheat the oven to 350°F (175°C). Line a baking sheet with parchment paper.
2. In a large bowl, mix almond flour, coconut sugar, baking soda, and salt.
3. Add melted coconut oil, egg, grated ginger, and vanilla extract. Stir until well combined.
4. Scoop tablespoon-sized balls of dough onto the prepared baking sheet.
5. Flatten each ball slightly with the back of a spoon.
6. Bake for 10-12 minutes, or until golden brown.
7. Allow to cool before serving.

Tips:

- Add a pinch of cinnamon for extra warmth.
- Store in an airtight container for up to a week.

Vanilla and Pecan Ice Cream

Portions: 6

Ingredients:

- 2 cups coconut milk
- 1/2 cup maple syrup
- 1 teaspoon vanilla extract
- 1/2 cup pecans, chopped

Preparation Time: 10 minutes + freezing time

Nutritional Information (per serving):

Calories	Carbohydrates	Protein	Fat	Fiber	Sugar	Sodium
200 kcal	18 g	2 g	14 g	2 g	16 g	15 mg

Instructions:

1. In a bowl, mix coconut milk, maple syrup, and vanilla extract.
2. Pour the mixture into an ice cream maker and churn according to the manufacturer's instructions.
3. Add chopped pecans in the last few minutes of churning.
4. Transfer to a container and freeze until firm, about 2-4 hours.
5. Serve scoops of ice cream in bowls.

Tips:

- Toast the pecans for extra flavor.
- Serve with fresh berries or a drizzle of chocolate sauce.

Peach and Raspberry Crumble

Portions: 6

Ingredients:

- 4 ripe peaches, sliced
- 1 cup raspberries
- 1/2 cup almond flour
- 1/2 cup oats
- 1/4 cup coconut sugar
- 1/4 cup coconut oil, melted
- 1 teaspoon cinnamon

Preparation Time: 30 minutes

Nutritional Information (per serving):

Calories	Carbohydrates	Protein	Fat	Fiber	Sugar	Sodium
220 kcal	28 g	3 g	12 g	6 g	18 g	30 mg

Instructions:

1. Preheat the oven to 350°F (175°C).
2. In a large bowl, combine sliced peaches and raspberries.
3. In another bowl, mix almond flour, oats, coconut sugar, melted coconut oil, and cinnamon.
4. Place the fruit mixture in a baking dish and sprinkle the crumble topping evenly over the fruit.
5. Bake for 20-25 minutes, or until the topping is golden brown and the fruit is bubbling.
6. Allow to cool slightly before serving.

Tips:

- Serve with a scoop of vanilla ice cream or a dollop of yogurt.
- Use a mix of berries for a different flavor profile.

Date and Almond Bars

Pieces: 12

Ingredients:

- 1 cup pitted dates
- 1 cup almonds
- 1/4 cup almond butter
- 1/4 cup shredded coconut
- 1 tablespoon chia seeds

Preparation Time: 15 minutes + chilling time

Nutritional Information (per serving):

Calories	Carbohydrates	Protein	Fat	Fiber	Sugar	Sodium
150 kcal	18 g	3 g	8 g	4 g	15 g	5 mg

Instructions:

1. In a food processor, blend pitted dates and almonds until a sticky dough forms.
2. Add almond butter, shredded coconut, and chia seeds. Pulse until well combined.
3. Press the mixture into a lined baking dish.
4. Refrigerate for at least 1 hour, or until firm.
5. Cut into bars and serve.

Tips:

- Store in the fridge for up to a week.
- Add dark chocolate chips for a sweet twist.

Pineapple and Coconut Cheesecake

Portions: 8

Ingredients:

- 1 cup raw cashews, soaked overnight
- 1/2 cup coconut cream
- 1/4 cup maple syrup
- 1/2 cup pineapple chunks
- 1/4 cup shredded coconut
- 1 teaspoon vanilla extract
- 1/2 cup almond flour (for the crust)
- 2 tablespoons coconut oil, melted (for the crust)

Preparation Time: 20 minutes + chilling time

Nutritional Information (per serving):

Calories	Carbohydrates	Protein	Fat	Fiber	Sugar	Sodium
250 kcal	18 g	4 g	18 g	3 g	10 g	20 mg

Instructions:

1. For the crust, mix almond flour and melted coconut oil. Press into the bottom of a springform pan.
2. In a blender, combine soaked cashews, coconut cream, maple syrup, pineapple chunks, shredded coconut, and vanilla extract until smooth.
3. Pour the mixture over the crust.
4. Refrigerate for at least 4 hours, or until set.
5. Serve chilled, garnished with extra pineapple and shredded coconut.

Tips:

- Use a mix of tropical fruits for a varied flavor.
- Top with a drizzle of honey or coconut flakes.

Smoothie

Green Goddess Smoothie

Portions: 2

Ingredients:

- 1 cup kale leaves
- 1/2 avocado
- 1 banana
- 1 cup unsweetened almond milk
- 1 tablespoon chia seeds
- 1 tablespoon honey (optional)

Preparation Time: 5 minutes

Nutritional Information (per serving):

Calories	Carbohydrates	Protein	Fat	Fiber	Sugar	Sodium
180 kcal	28 g	3 g	8 g	7 g	12 g	50 mg

Instructions:

1. Add all ingredients to a blender.
2. Blend until smooth.
3. Pour into glasses and serve immediately.

Tips:

- Add a handful of spinach for extra greens.
- Use frozen banana for a thicker consistency.

Red Beet Reviver

Portions: 2

Ingredients:

- 1 small beet, peeled and chopped
- 1 apple, cored and chopped
- 1/2 cup carrots, chopped
- 1 cup orange juice
- 1 tablespoon lemon juice

Preparation Time: 5 minutes

Nutritional Information (per serving):

Calories	Carbohydrates	Protein	Fat	Fiber	Sugar	Sodium
120 kcal	28 g	2 g	0 g	5 g	20 g	30 mg

Instructions:

1. Add all ingredients to a blender.
2. Blend until smooth.
3. Pour into glasses and serve immediately.

Tips:

- Add a piece of ginger for a spicy kick.
- Use chilled ingredients for a refreshing drink.

Tropical Turmeric Cleanser

Portions: 2

Ingredients:

- 1 cup pineapple chunks
- 1 orange, peeled
- 1/2 banana
- 1/2 teaspoon turmeric powder
- 1 cup coconut water

Preparation Time: 5 minutes

Nutritional Information (per serving):

Calories	Carbohydrates	Protein	Fat	Fiber	Sugar	Sodium
110 kcal	26 g	1 g	0 g	3 g	20 g	40 mg

Instructions:

1. Add all ingredients to a blender.
2. Blend until smooth.
3. Pour into glasses and serve immediately.

Tips:

- Add a pinch of black pepper to enhance turmeric absorption.
- Use frozen pineapple for a cooler drink.

Berry Alkaline Boost

Portions: 2

Ingredients:

- 1 cup mixed berries (strawberries, blueberries, raspberries)
- 1/2 cucumber, peeled and chopped
- 1/2 cup spinach
- 1 tablespoon chia seeds
- 1 cup coconut water

Preparation Time: 5 minutes

Nutritional Information (per serving):

Calories	Carbohydrates	Protein	Fat	Fiber	Sugar	Sodium
90 kcal	22 g	2 g	2 g	7 g	12 g	35 mg

Instructions:

1. Add all ingredients to a blender.
2. Blend until smooth.
3. Pour into glasses and serve immediately.

Tips:

- Add a few mint leaves for a refreshing twist.
- Use frozen berries for a thicker smoothie.

Minty Melon Mixer

Portions: 2

Ingredients:

- 1 cup watermelon chunks
- 1/2 cucumber, peeled and chopped
- 1/2 cup fresh mint leaves
- 1 tablespoon lime juice
- 1 cup cold water

Preparation Time: 5 minutes

Nutritional Information (per serving):

Calories	Carbohydrates	Protein	Fat	Fiber	Sugar	Sodium
60 kcal	14 g	1 g	0 g	2 g	10 g	10 mg

Instructions:

1. Add all ingredients to a blender.
2. Blend until smooth.
3. Pour into glasses and serve immediately.

Tips:

- Use sparkling water for a fizzy variation.
- Garnish with additional mint leaves.

Carrot Ginger Zing

Portions: 2

Ingredients:

- 1 cup carrots, chopped
- 1 apple, cored and chopped
- 1/2 inch fresh ginger, peeled
- 1 cup orange juice
- 1/2 cup ice cubes

Preparation Time: 5 minutes

Nutritional Information (per serving):

Calories	Carbohydrates	Protein	Fat	Fiber	Sugar	Sodium
100 kcal	24 g	1 g	0 g	4 g	18 g	20 mg

Instructions:

1. Add all ingredients to a blender.
2. Blend until smooth.
3. Pour into glasses and serve immediately.

Tips:

- Add a pinch of cinnamon for extra warmth.
- Use chilled orange juice for a cooler drink.

Creamy Avocado Dream

Portions: 2

Ingredients:

- 1 avocado, peeled and pitted
- 1 banana
- 1 cup unsweetened almond milk
- 1 tablespoon honey (optional)
- 1/2 teaspoon vanilla extract

Preparation Time: 5 minutes

Nutritional Information (per serving):

Calories	Carbohydrates	Protein	Fat	Fiber	Sugar	Sodium
200 kcal	24 g	3 g	12 g	7 g	12 g	40 mg

Instructions:

1. Add all ingredients to a blender.
2. Blend until smooth.
3. Pour into glasses and serve immediately.

Tips:

- Use frozen banana for a thicker consistency.
- Add a tablespoon of cocoa powder for a chocolate version.

Sweet Potato Pie Smoothie

Portions: 2

Ingredients:

- 1/2 cup cooked sweet potato
- 1 banana
- 1 cup unsweetened almond milk
- 1 tablespoon maple syrup
- 1/2 teaspoon cinnamon
- 1/4 teaspoon nutmeg

Preparation Time: 5 minutes

Nutritional Information (per serving):

Calories	Carbohydrates	Protein	Fat	Fiber	Sugar	Sodium
150 kcal	30 g	2 g	3 g	4 g	16 g	45 mg

Instructions:

1. Add all ingredients to a blender.
2. Blend until smooth.
3. Pour into glasses and serve immediately.

Tips:

- Use chilled sweet potato for a cooler drink.
- Add a dollop of whipped coconut cream for extra indulgence.

Pineapple Parsley Punch

Portions: 2

Ingredients:

- 1 cup pineapple chunks
- 1/2 cup parsley leaves
- 1/2 cucumber, peeled and chopped
- 1 cup coconut water
- 1 tablespoon lime juice

Preparation Time: 5 minutes

Nutritional Information (per serving):

Calories	Carbohydrates	Protein	Fat	Fiber	Sugar	Sodium
70 kcal	15 g	2 g	0 g	3 g	10 g	25 mg

Instructions:

1. Add all ingredients to a blender.
2. Blend until smooth.
3. Pour into glasses and serve immediately.

Tips:

- Add a few mint leaves for extra freshness.
- Use frozen pineapple for a thicker smoothie.

Spicy Cinnamon Apple Detox

Portions: 2

Ingredients:

- 1 apple, cored and chopped
- 1/2 cup carrots, chopped
- 1/2 teaspoon cinnamon
- 1 tablespoon lemon juice
- 1 cup water
- 1/2 cup ice cubes

Preparation Time: 5 minutes

Nutritional Information (per serving):

Calories	Carbohydrates	Protein	Fat	Fiber	Sugar	Sodium
80 kcal	20 g	1 g	0 g	4 g	15 g	10 mg

Instructions:

1. Add all ingredients to a blender.
2. Blend until smooth.
3. Pour into glasses and serve immediately.

Tips:

- Use chilled water for a cooler drink.
- Add a pinch of cayenne pepper for extra spice.

QR-CODE MEAL PLAN

To help you get started on your journey toward optimal health, we've included a QR code at the end of this book.

Scan it to download a comprehensive 60-day meal plan tailored to Dr. Sebi's alkaline diet principles.

Your feedback is invaluable to us. Please consider leaving a review to share your experience and help others discover the benefits of Dr. Sebi's Cookbook. Your thoughts and insights are greatly appreciated!

www.ingramcontent.com/pod-product-compliance
Lightning Source LLC
LaVergne TN
LVHW060202080526
838202LV00052B/4184